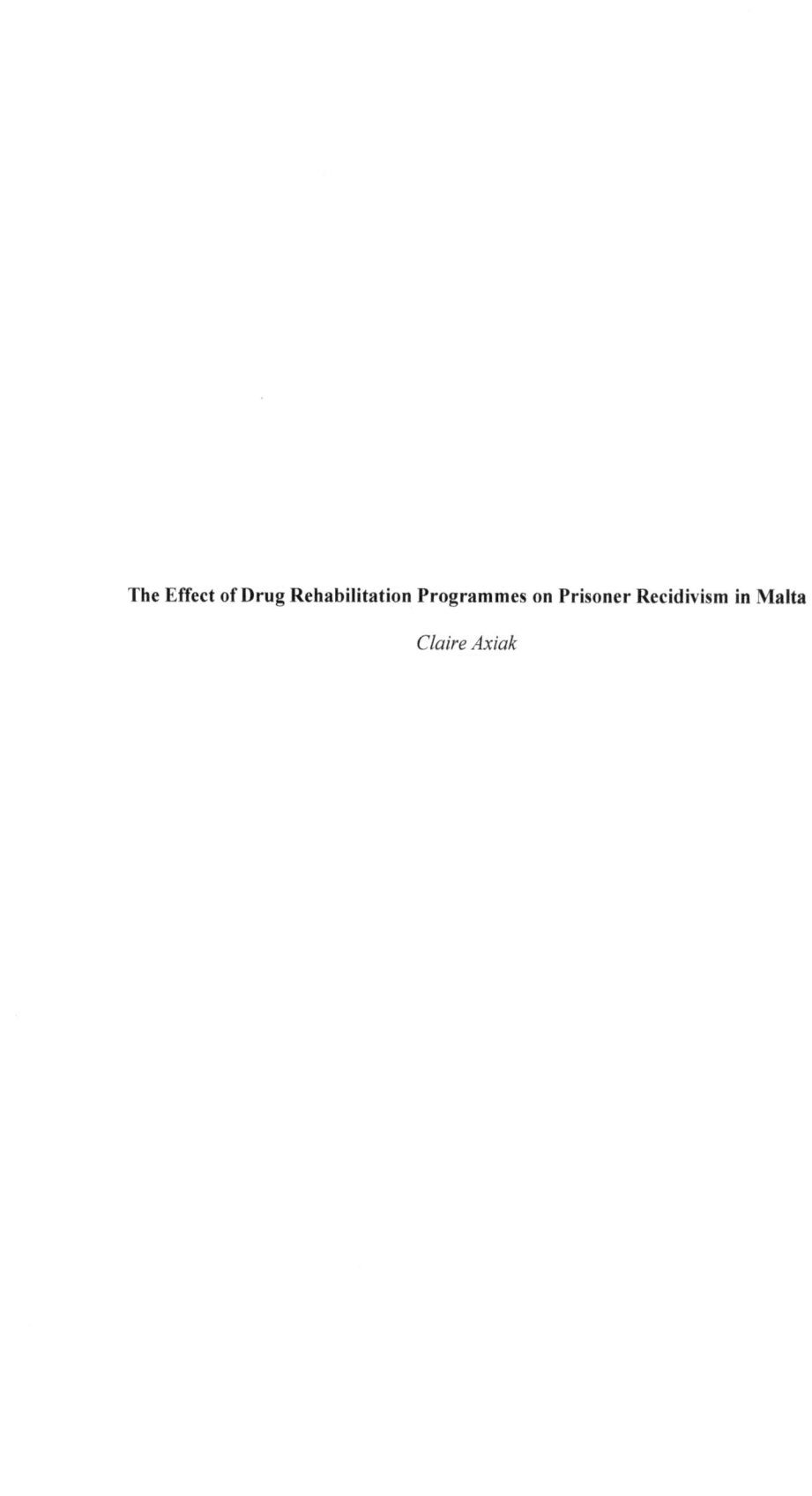

The Effect of Drug Rehabilitation Programmes on Prisoner Recidivism in Malta

Claire Axiak

Preface

Drug abuse is a serious social phenomenon in Malta with the prevalence amongst adults reaching 14% amongst those aged 18-24 years. Besides the well-known harmful effects on the person, substance misuse may also have serious repercussions on society due to the strain on public finances spent on medical interventions, court proceedings, production losses and payment of benefits. However the argument for financing prison inmate programmes (PiPs) is compelling in light of various studies establishing the positive effect of such treatment, especially based on the therapeutic community (TC) model, on reducing recidivism. This study examined the impact of TC PiPs on recidivism amongst inmates released from prison between 2005-2008 including the effect of completion of such programs on recidivism as against dropping out. Two comparison groups of inmates who did not attend a PiP or who attended in the past were included in the study. A number of statistical tests including chi-square tests, independent t-tests, Fisher's Exact Tests, ANOVA and generalized linear models (glm) with a logit link function were employed in the analysis. Although results did not reject the null hypotheses and PiP participation was not determined to be a significant predictor of recidivism, a number of interesting findings were made. The author discussed the study's limitations including those that may have influenced the results and also made recommendations for future research and changes in policy.

Dedication

To Victor, Kristina and Luke

Acknowledgements

This study would not have been possible without the support and encouragement I received from my family during the long hours spent researching the topic. Nor would it have been possible without the foresight, determination and thankless initiative shown by Major Vince Vassallo, Amadeo Scerri and Joanne Battistino in compiling and regularly maintaining inmate data at the Corradino Correctional Facility. I have benefited greatly from the mentoring of Consultant Dr. Joseph Spiteri for whom I am truly indebted. I would also like to thank Dr. Neville Calleja (Director at Department of Health Information & Research) for his immense help and assistance with the statistics used in this study. Last but not least I would like to thank Mgr. Victor Grech (Director of Caritas Malta), Jesmond Schembri (Operations Director of Sedqa) and Abraham Zammit (Acting Director of Corradino Correctional Facility) for their endorsement and support of this dissertation.

Table of Contents

List of Tables

List of Tables in Appendices

Appendix B

Chapter 1: Introduction

Background

The problem of substance misuse in Malta has been stated and overstated for many years to such an extent that at times it becomes rather unclear whether public perception is actually a misguided state of affairs brought about by extensive and regular media exposure to the problem. Unfortunately, official statistics paint a rather grim picture of the situation and all but confirm that drug abuse is indeed a serious social phenomenon in the Maltese Islands. According to the Lifestyle Survey 2007 (National Statistics Office (NSO), 2009), the prevalence of illicit substance misuse amongst adults during the 12 months immediately preceding the survey was about 3.2%., with a peak of use (14%) registered amongst those aged 18 to 24 years.

Regular studies have been conducted by the European School Survey Project on Alcohol and Other Drugs (ESPAD) amongst student populations (aged between 15 and 16 years) in Europe (Hibell, Guttormsson, Ahlström, Balakireva, Bjarnason, Kokkevi & Kraus, 2012). Malta rates favourably in relation to other European countries with regard to lifetime prevalence estimates of cannabis (10% vs. 17%) and equally with regard to other illicit drugs such as ecstasy, cocaine and heroin (6% vs. 6%). However, lifetime use of inhalants is much higher than the European average (14% vs. 9%).

The primary drug of use amongst persons undergoing treatment is heroin (80%), followed by cocaine (11%) and cannabis (5%) in contrast to the situation in the majority of European countries where cannabis (50%-90%) continues to be the main illicit drug of choice (European Monitoring Centre for Drugs and Drug Addiction (EMCDDA), 2011; EMCDDA, 2012). A rather worrying statistic is that Malta has the third highest annual prevalence rate of opioid use in Europe (6.1 cases per 1,000 population aged 15 to 64) which compares unfavourably with the average prevalence (between 3.6 to 4.4 cases per 1,000 population aged 15 to 64) in Europe (EMCDDA, 2012).

In the Diagnostic and Statistical Manual of Mental Disorders – Fourth Edition, Text Revision of the American Psychiatric Association (DSM–IV–TR (2000) 4th ed., text rev.), substance abuse is defined as "a maladaptive pattern of substance use leading to clinically significant impairment or distress" as manifested by the fulfilment of one or more of specific criteria within a 12-month period, including failure to carry out "major role obligations at work, school or home", recurrent substance use in physically dangerous situations, legal problems (e.g. drink-driving arrests) and continued substance misuse in spite of recurring social or personal problems that may be caused by the effects of the substance. Amongst the changes seen in DSM-5, the disease categories for substance abuse and dependence have been eliminated and replaced with a new "addictions and related disorders" category including substance use disorders with each drug identified in its own category. The 10th revision of the International Statistical Classification of Diseases and Related Health Problems (ICD-10) on the other hand refers to "harmful use" (rather than "substance or drug abuse") as "a pattern of psychoactive substance use that is causing damage to health" where the damage may be either physical (e.g. hepatitis following injection of drugs) or mental (e.g. depressive episodes secondary to heavy alcohol intake). Undesirable social consequences in isolation are not sufficient to justify a diagnosis of harmful use in ICD-10 although they are mentioned as a common occurrence.

Besides the well-known harmful effects on one's health and welfare, substance misuse may have serious repercussions on society at large not least due to the strain on public finances spent on medical interventions, loss of production, payment of state benefits due to social cases and unemployment, court proceedings, etc. Unfortunately there is no available information on the national drug-related public expenditure so one can only speculate on the possible impact of drug abuse on the public coffers. It is known however that the expenditure incurred between the years 2008 and 2010 in connection with the operation and running of the three prison inmate programmes (PIPs) amounted to almost two million euro (Maltese Parliament, 2011).

Nonetheless, even during these challenging times of financial crisis, the argument for financing effective drug treatment programs is compelling not least because research has shown that prison-based treatment, especially programs based on the therapeutic community (TC) model have a positive effect on reducing reincarceration (Inciardi, Martin, Butzin, Hooper & Harrison, 1997; Knight, Simpson & Hiller, 1999; Prendergast, Podus, Chang & Urada, 2002). Also, the cost-effectiveness of substance abuse treatment for offenders is justifiable in large part because of the reduced criminal activity associated with the cessation of substance use and abuse (Substance Abuse and Mental Health Services Administration (SAMHSA), 2005).

Maltese law regulating drugs consists in the Dangerous Drugs Ordinance (1939) which deals with narcotics (e.g. opium, cannabis, cocaine, etc.) and in the Medical and Kindred Professions Ordinance (1901) which deals with psychotropic drugs. Punishments for drug-related offences are invariably custodial in nature although fines for minor misdemeanours may be imposed in lieu of incarceration. For instance anyone convicted of simple possession in the Court of Magistrates is liable to imprisonment for a period between 3 to 12 months and/or to a fine ranging between €470 and €2,350. On the other hand possession indicating that drugs were not for the offender's sole and exclusive use (including any forms of cultivation) carries very harsh sanctions including life imprisonment. At present Maltese law does not provide for sanctions that are not criminal in nature although the imminent establishment of a Drugs Court would change this scenario and no doubt alleviate some of the burden carried by the Corradino Correctional Facility.

A common and founded perception amongst the public is that a considerable proportion of crimes committed locally, especially theft, are attributable to drug users. Indeed, it has been reported (Gellel, Olivari D'Emanuele & Muscat, 2011) that during the

9

year 2010, out of a total of 731 inmates at the Corradino Correctional Facility, 37% were serving a custodial sentence for drug-related offences. More damningly, after being tested, 223 inmates (representing 30.5% of the inmate population) tested positive during 2010 for opiates, cocaine, cannabis or a mix of two or all drug types although this data does not indicate whether testing was carried out on admission or during the stay at Corradino Correctional Facility. Inmates testing positive are penalised in accordance to Prison Regulations and are not charged in Court.

Corradino Correctional Facility is the only correctional institution in Malta and houses all people who have been remanded in custody or convicted by the local courts. Inmates (on drug-related offences) who satisfy a number of criteria and pass an assessment by the Prison Substance Abuse Assessment Board are given permission to attend a prison inmate program for the rest of their custodial sentence. These criteria include, serving a sentence of not less than 6 months but not more than 2 years, regular good conduct and absence of mental illness or mental disorders although in all cases exceptions are considered.

There are three prison inmate programmes currently in operation in Malta under the supervision of the Prison Board. These are operated by Caritas (a voluntary treatment provider which receives partial financial support from the Government), the Substance Abuse Therapeutic Unit ("SATU") which is prison based and falls under the responsibility of the Ministry of Justice and Home Affairs, and the Santa Maria Programme run by SEDQA (the national agency against drugs and alcohol abuse forming part of the Ministry of Education, Employment and the Family) which since 1999 began accepting referrals from prison.

Although they differ in regime and intervention approach, these residential programmes are based on the TC model and the residential phase corresponds to the period of the remaining prison sentence. Participation is on a voluntary basis and prisoners who are eligible may indicate a preference for a programme of their choice.

The number of residents following drug rehabilitation outside of prison varies constantly. During 2010, 34 residents followed drug treatment in an outside agency. In 2011, 8 inmates enrolled with SATU, 13 with Sedqa and 8 with Caritas. The majority of clients in treatment are heroin users (85%).

Notwithstanding the potentially crucial benefits to inmates and society at large and the significant expenditure incurred, the use and impact of these pre-release programmes is not monitored in an extensive or systematic manner. According to the Corradino Correctional Facility many prisoners do not choose to enrol for the pre-release programme and of those that do, many do not finish the programme for a number of reasons ranging from lack of commitment to breach of regulations, and thus return to the Corradino Correctional Facility to serve the remainder of their custodial sentence. More importantly, no study has ever been undertaken which examines the efficacy of these programmes in preventing reoffending.

While there is ample evidence that shows that a significant proportion of prisoners at the Corradino Correctional Facility are drug-related offenders, out of which, another sizeable proportion test positive for opiates, cocaine, cannabis or a mix of two or all drug types, the effectiveness of prison-inmate programmes in reducing recidivism of inmates at the Corradino Correctional Facility is not known since no study has ever been undertaken to examine such possible correlation.

Studies undertaken abroad show that where there is no effective treatment for drug abusers who offend, the likelihood is that a good number of the latter will reoffend. Multiple studies also indicate that such offenders reoffend much more than those offenders who do not abuse of drugs (Bureau of Justice Statistics (BJS), 1995; Gendreau, Little & Goggin, 1996;

11

Horney, Osgood & Marshall, 1995; MacKenzie, Browning, Skroban & Smith, 1999). It is thus not a coincidence that the period of imprisonment is one of the most crucial periods where intervention is required to stop the cycle of drug abuse and criminality.

In a recent meta-analytic study Mitchell, Wilson & MacKenzie (2007) postulated that the most reliable evidence of the effectiveness of treatment for the prevention of reoffending comes from evaluations of prison-inmate programmes conducted in Therapeutic Communities. The authors found evidence that such programmes demonstrated on a regular basis a decline in recidivism and drug relapse after release from prison. In their literature review, it was revealed that the majority of Residential Programmes are founded on the therapeutic community model, as is the case locally. The authors concluded that there is not enough knowledge and awareness as to which specific parts of treatment programs are the most important or which combinations are most effective in preventing reoffending.

Purpose of the study

The main purpose of this study is to determine the efficacy, or otherwise, of drug rehabilitation programmes (i.e. the prison inmate programmes offered by Caritas, Sedqa and the Substance Abuse Therapeutic Unit) in reducing recidivism among inmates at the Corradino Correctional Facility. It also attempts to examine whether completion of such programs (as against participating and dropping out) has any effect on recidivism rates and seeks to identify predictors and risk factors for reoffending with implications for future risk management.

Research design

The present study is a quasi-experimental retrospective cohort study designed to determine the impact of prison inmate programmes on recidivism amongst inmates at the

12

Corradino Correctional Facility. Existing data consisting in electronic files maintained and

kept at the Corradino Correctional Facility by dedicated individuals was collected. These files

contained extensive information on inmates admitted to the Corradino Correctional Facility

since 1946 including date of birth, age at admission, occupational status, type of conviction

and date of sentences. Other files contained information with regard to participation in prison

inmate programmes, psychiatric treatment pre-admission, psychiatric treatment post-

admission and substance-replacement therapy in the Corradino Correctional Facility. The

latter files were compiled on inmates admitted to the Corradino Correctional Facility in the

last decade or so. Data compiled by administrators of the three prison inmate programs was

also collected. This consisted of information in relation to completion or non-completion of

the programs.

No treatment was involved and no experimental procedures involving human

subjects were carried out.

Data was gathered on three groups of inmates having a history of substance abuse all

of whom were released from the Corradino Correctional Facility between 2005 and 2008.

One group consisted of all inmates who did not participate in any prison inmate program

during the time spent in prison for a conviction that ended between 2005 and 2008 but who

had participated in such programmes in the past. Another group consisted of all inmates who

never participated in any prison inmate programme. The third group consisted of all inmates

who participated in at least one of the prison inmate programmes during the time spent in

prison for a conviction that ended between 2005 and 2008.

Recidivism data was collected and analysed using the existing data. Possible predictor

variables including age on admission, sex, occupation, in-prison psychiatric treatment, in-

prison substance-replacement therapy, the number of prior incarcerations and age on first

13

conviction were available in the collected data and were thus included in the analysis. However there was a lack of availability of data concerning possible confounding variables after release from Corradino Correctional Facility and moreover such data could not be collected since the research design did not include contact with subjects

Research Questions and Hypotheses

Research Question 1: Are offenders with substance-use disorder who participate in a prison inmate program less likely to reoffend than offenders who did not participate in any such program?

Null Hypothesis 1: Offenders with substance-use disorder who participate in a prison inmate program are not less likely to reoffend than offenders who did not participate in any such program.

Alternate Hypothesis 1: Offenders with substance-use disorder who participate in a prison inmate program are less likely to reoffend than offenders who did not participate in any such program.

Research Question 2: Are offenders with substance-use disorder who participate in a particular prison inmate program and complete such program less likely to reoffend than offenders who participate in but drop out of any one of the other prison inmate programmes?

Null Hypothesis 2: Offenders with substance-use disorder who participate in and complete a particular prison inmate program are not less likely to reoffend than offenders who participate in and drop out of any one of the other prison inmate programmes.

Alternate Hypothesis 2: Offenders with substance-use disorder who participate in and complete a particular prison inmate program are less likely to reoffend than offenders who participate in and drop out of any one of the other prison inmate programmes

14

Definition of recidivism

Recidivism in this study was defined as any offence committed after release from the Corradino Correctional Facility between 2005 and 2008 for which the offender has been given a conviction by the Maltese Courts necessitating a custodial sentence and re-entry into prison. Therefore convictions resulting in a conditional discharge, probation or suspended sentences were not taken into consideration. Release from prison was defined as an unconditional release from incarceration, thus not including release on bail. The word "reoffending" is used interchangeably with "recidivating" for the purpose of this study although they are technically distinct from each other as explained in the final chapter.

Expected findings

It was expected that the findings of this study would be consistent with previous studies, discussed in the literature review, that prison inmate programs reduce the rate of recidivism and that inmates who go on to complete such a program are less likely to recidivate when compared to those that enter but do not complete the program.

Chapter 2: The Prison Inmate Programmes

Therapeutic Community Based Treatment

Therapeutic communities are highly structured intensive residential programmes of a relatively long duration that deal with the underlying causes of drug addiction in order to treat the client who is guided throughout a transitional period of well-being. The first TC was established in the US in 1962 and prison-based TCs proliferated in the years that followed until the early 1980s. They were indeed the main type of addiction treatment provided in the prison sitting in the States. Due to budget constraints and prison overcrowding, a significant number closed down in the early eighties (Martin, Butzin, Saum & Inciardi, 1999) but the model was adapted and remerged in the late eighties to become once again the principal type of drug treatment in the prison environment eventually spreading to Europe (Inciardi & Martin, 1993). Studies of these prison-based TCs began to reveal a mostly positive outcome on recidivism rates of inmates convicted of drug-related offences. (Griffith, Hiller, Knight, & Simpson, 1999; Knight et al. 1999; Martin et al. 1999; Pearson & Lipton, 1999).

The US Government recognised that the success of prison-based TCs in reducing criminality would be cost-effective and lead to substantial savings for the public coffers (Martin et al. 1999; SAMHSA, 2005). It was therefore no surprise when in 1994 the US Congress established the Residential Substance Abuse Treatment (RSAT) Program under the Violent Crime Control and Law Enforcement Act of 1994. RSAT was intended to provide financial support to correctional facilities across the US to enable them to develop, maintain and implement in-prison substance abuse treatment programs. This was seen as the culmination of the US's recognition of the effectiveness of prison-based TCs. Today, programs that are funded by RSAT are typically based on the therapeutic community model.

The raison d'être of TCs is that the individual who suffers from drug addiction has various aspects of his functioning that are affected by the substance misuse including cognitive and behavioural issues. Therefore the individual's addiction problem should be treated by dealing with the whole spectrum of issues that such individual faces in his everyday life. The main goals of treatment in TC based treatment involve a radical change in the client's lifestyle including moderation, self-restraint, abstinence, removal of anti-social behaviour and fostering of pro-social values and conduct (Prendergast, Farabee & Cartier, 2001). The client is handled responsibility for taking control over the choices he makes and decisions he takes in his life. Cognitive-behavioural techniques that change maladaptive thoughts and behaviour may also be incorporated into treatment (Taxman & Bouffard, 2002).

Typically, clients entering the community have a recent history of worsening educational skills, family relationships and social functioning due to their addiction. Rehabilitation through the reestablishment of such skills and values is therefore paramount. Severe problems such as multiple addictions, mental health issues and criminal conduct are also dealt with. The key characteristic of TCs when compared with other forms of addiction treatments is the structured social environment often consisting of a rigid hierarchy with separate stages of treatment and different roles carrying different privileges and responsibilities. Manual work may be incorporated in TCs and in such case is part of the treatment itself.

In Malta there are a number of TC based treatments offered to drug addicts, a number of whom are open exclusively to inmates at the Corradino Correctional Facility such as the three prison inmate programmes analysed in this study. Such programmes house clients in units that are physically separate and distinct from the potentially negative influences of prison. Inmates are heavily involved in running the community such as for instance by

17

leading treatment sessions, supervising and/or monitoring other residents for compliance with regulations and resolving disputes. Inmates are also challenged and confronted with regard to any anti-social conduct or harmful beliefs that they might have. The residential stage of the programmes varies according to the remaining period of the sentence of the resident.

Applications for admission are made on a voluntary basis by inmates. The procedure is anything but straightforward and one has to be selected on a unanimous basis by the Prisoners' Substance Abuse Assessment Board, an independent board that includes representatives from Sedqa, Caritas and SATU, the Director of Prisons, the rehabilitation manager, prison psychologists and the doctor in charge of SATU. First of all the inmate must have been in prison for a period of not less than six months, his or her sentence must be one not exceeding two years and he/she must not have any pending criminal proceedings. A rigorous process is then carried out including tests that assess the motivation of the prisoner and the severity of his or her addiction. The board ultimately decides whether the inmate fits within the set parameters and in that case informs him or her that the application has been successful. It is also the board's decision as to which program will be followed by the prisoner.

The Substance Abuse Therapeutic Unit (SATU)

Formerly known as the Substance Abuse Assessment Unit (SAAU), SATU is operated by the Department of Correctional Services and is situated in Mtahleb. The prison-inmate rehabilitation program was developed in 1996 and has made leaps and bounds over the years to become a very important tool in the rehabilitation of inmates at the Corradino Correctional Facility having a history of substance misuse. The mission statement of SATU states that drug addictions have a multitude of predisposing interrelated factors that can ultimately be changed through the inmate's sheer will and determination to follow the

18

treatment program to its end. Inmates suffering from dual diagnosis are also eligible for the program.

As is the case in the other prison inmate programmes, prisoners enter and stay in SATU out of their own free will and volition but can only stay if they adhere to a strict code of ethics and rules.

Prisoners participate in various programs designed to help them change their ways and restore their values in time for their return to society. These programs include self-help groups, psychotherapy groups, motivational therapeutic group sessions, individual and family counselling sessions, life skills sessions, adult education groups and couple therapy sessions. During the motivational therapeutic group sessions, inmates are challenged and confronted by professionals such as psychotherapists about their behaviour. The aim of these sessions is to encourage and sustain drug abstention. Family sessions are also an important component of the program whereby the inmate's closed relatives and friends are invited to attend and assist in the recovery process.

Inmates are also required to work during the residential stage and to divide and organise work amongst themselves (such as daily chores, maintenance jobs and technical duties) in a hierarchical fashion using the network principle. They are also assigned tasks that reflect the progress of their individual stay with increasing responsibilities and privileges. A rigid daily schedule encompassing rest breaks, work, therapeutic sessions and leisure has to be adhered to by each resident. This rigid structure is intended to counteract the self-indulgent and destructive lifestyle that is so typically associated with addiction.

The prison inmates program is made up of three main phase. During the first phase the inmate is introduced to and is required to acclimatise himself or herself to the rules and requirements of the program and to face up to his or her specific issues and personality

19

problems. Motivation and support is given with the aim of encouraging the individual to start changing his or her behaviour. During the next phase, the inmate is expected to have started appreciating his or her power to take decisions that reverse the negative trends that have taken hold of his or her life. Education and therapy groups are aimed at fostering this new-found belief that will hopefully remain with the inmate throughout his or her life.

During the last three to six months of his or her sentence, the inmate is sent out to work on prison leave. This experience of community life outside of prison is then shared with his or her fellow inmates upon return to the unit in the evening. After release, a five-year plan that is aimed at following up the inmate's progress out of prison is offered.

Komunità Santa Marija (Sedqa)

Agenzija Sedqa operates a highly structured residential programme at Hal Farrug for drug addicts known as "Komunita' Santa Marija" part of which is open to prison inmates. It is constituted of a Unit Leader, a Programme Coordinator, a number of specialised Care Workers teachers, priests and volunteers. As is the case in SATU, the aim is to foster discipline and a sense of structure in the inmate's lifestyle that balances the haphazard and destructive influences in his or her life. Particular emphasis is placed on psychotherapy to assist clients in addressing their internal conflicts and underlying causes that may have led to their dependence on drugs. Family involvement, education and spiritual needs are also catered for so as to contribute to a holistic way of treating the client.

The program is divided into various stages: merhba (welcome), formazzjoni (formation), responsabilta' (responsibility), sfida (challenge) and aftercare. Between one stage and the next the inmate faces increasingly difficult challenges as well as an increase in privileges and duties. The "sfida" phase is semi-residential while the "after-care" phrase

20

involves six months of follow-up scrutiny and monthly progress group-meetings. Individuals who complete the program in its entirety, that is, the residential phase, the semi-residential phase and the after-care phase, are candidates for graduation.

New Hope Prison Inmate Programme (Caritas)

This programme, operated by Caritas and financed by the Ministry for Justice, Dialogue and the Family, is housed in Bahar ic-Caghaq. It is largely similar to the other residential program also operated by Caritas in San Blas and indeed is an offshoot of such programme. The service addresses the client from a spiritual, socio-legal, physical and psychological aspect and it also involves relatives and individuals who are close to the inmate as it is felt that the latter actually become part of the problem or indeed were its cause in the first place.

The programme consists of four stages: the residential phase (corresponding to the remaining period of the prison sentence), the semi-residential phase, the re-entry phase and the aftercare phase. During the residential phase which lasts approximately eight months inmates are introduced to the tools that are required to start building a new life once the program is completed. This phase has three major tests or stages – every 2/3 months– each of which the inmate must successfully complete in order to progress to the next stage. A process of evaluation of the inmate's conduct and progress throughout this phase is carried out. In the semi-residential phase, inmates are given assistance for reintegration back into the community such as for instance by searching for potential employment opportunities and attendance of vocational training and courses. The re-entry phase, as its name suggests, prepares inmates who have completed successfully the residential phase for their return to life outside the program and outside prison. Inmates participate in both group sessions and one-

21

to-one sessions intended to further their self-development. After a minimum of 6-8 months from the completion of the residential phase, an inmate graduates from the programme. After graduation, support for maintenance of drug abstinence is given through fortnightly group meetings that are attended by both inmates, their families and past graduates that lend a helping hand.

The problem of retention

The majority of inmates who enter treatment do not complete the programme and are sent back to the Corradino Correctional Facility. By way of example, with regard to Komunita' Santa Marija (Sedqa), in 2007 the percentage of persons who completed the programme amounted to 16.6%. This went up to 24.2% in 2008 and decreased to 21.6% in 2009 (Foundation for Social Welfare Services (FSWS), 2011). Most often, inmates drop out due to infringement of the rules, lack of progress or sheer unwillingness and lack of determination to commit to the strict tasks.

In this study, one of the three groups that were studied consisted solely of all inmates who participated in at least one of the prison inmate programmes during the time spent in prison for a conviction that ended between 2005 and 2008. Within this group (consisting of 105 inmates), 32 inmates participated in the TC program operated by SATU, 35 inmates participated in the program operated by Sedqa and 38 inmates participated in the program operated by Caritas. Within the group of 32 inmates that went to SATU 15 inmates completed the program (i.e. 47%), within the group of 35 inmates that went to Sedqa 14 completed and graduated from the program (i.e. 40%) whilst within the group of 38 inmates that went to Caritas 18 inmates completed and graduated from the program (i.e. 47%)

22

This problem of retention raises the question of whether the benefits of the relative programs are being received in their entirety. This notwithstanding, the literature review shows that despite high drop-out rates, therapeutic communities have proved to be effective in reducing recidivism (Dekel, Benbenishty & Amran, 2004). Various studies, including this study, have incorporated both persons who graduate and others who drop out prematurely. Interestingly, retention has been found to be an important predictor of long-term success (DeLeon, 2000; Quinones, Doyle, Sheffet & Louria, 1979). Prendergast et al. (2004) found that while inmates who participated in a prison inmate program, regardless of completion or not, reoffended substantially less than the comparison group, when the treatment group was subdivided into smaller groups, the program completers were the least likely to reoffend.

In view of such studies, it was deemed important by the author to carry out a comparison in recidivism rates between dropouts and completers. If there is a correlation between completion and less recidivism then a quantitative and qualitative research would be warranted to determine the factors that may possibly help an inmate to complete a program.

Chapter 3: Literature Review

The literature review is dominated by the United States' experience which is not surprising given that therapeutic communities originated in the United States. Multiple studies demonstrate that where there is no effective treatment for drug abusers who offend, the likelihood is that a good number of the latter will reoffend. They also indicate that such offenders reoffend much more than those offenders who do not abuse of drugs (Bureau of Justice Statistics 1995; Gendreau et al. 1996; Horney et al. 1995; MacKenzie et al. 1999). It is thus not a coincidence that the period of imprisonment is one of the most crucial periods where intervention is required to stop the cycle of drug abuse and criminality.

Effects of TC-based prison treatment on recidivism

The literature contains concrete evidence pointing towards the effectiveness of in-prison residential treatment that is based on the TC model on reducing reincarceration amongst inmates with a history of drug abuse and drug-related convictions. However a common point of criticism is that studies that demonstrate such effectiveness are methodologically weak. Moreover the benefits of such treatment in reducing drug relapse are still unclear at best.

In a meta-analytic study carried out by Mitchell et al. (2007) the authors examined the effectiveness of five types of prison-based drug treatment programs including TCs in reducing recidivism and drug use. This was done by a meta-analysis of the results collected from 66 published and unpublished studies on the subject. Reference was made to Pearson and Lipton who had already carried out a similar meta-analysis in 1999 by reviewing 30 experimental and quasi-experimental studies that had looked into the effectiveness of prison-based drug abuse programs between 1968 and 1996. This study revealed a number of

24

interesting findings chief amongst which was that in 6 out of 7 evaluations, inmates who

attended therapeutic-community based programs recidivated less than those who did not. The

overall mean-weighted effect size was 0.133 (p=0.025). The authors concluded that the

available evidence with regard to the effectiveness of such programs was indeed promising.

On their part, Mitchell et al.'s analytic review covered those studies that investigated

the impact of various forms of prison-based drug treatment given between 1980 and 2004 on

recidivism and drug relapse. The authors also found evidence that residential inmate

programmes based on therapeutic communities consistently showed post-release reductions

in recidivism though there were mixed results with regard to the effect on drug relapse. This

finding was consistent independently of any methodological variations or changes in sample

sizes or the specific features of the programmes. The authors analysed ten studies that had

gone into the relationship between residential therapeutic-community based programmes and

recidivism and found that these generated a mean odds ratio of 1.30 (95% Confidence

Interval 1.10–1.76) for recidivism outcomes thus proving the effectiveness of such programs

in that regard.

Interestingly, the association between participation in the programmes and lower rates

of recidivism remained strong irrespective of factors such as age, gender, type of offence and

coercion-based participation. This is outlined in Table 1.

Table 1

Odds ratios for offending by sample/treatment features

Coded feature	Mean ES	95% CI	k[a]
Age group of sample			
Adults	1.37*	1.18–1.60	27
Juveniles	1.47	0.89–2.43	2
Gender composition of sample			
All female	1.65*	1.14–2.39	6
Mixed (male and female)	1.23	0.84–1.79	4
All male	1.36*	1.13–1.64	18
Offender type			
Non-violent offenders	1.49*	1.24–1.79	15
Mixed (violent and non-violent)	1.28*	1.02–1.62	9
Mandatory aftercare			
No	1.31*	1.07–1.59	14
Yes	1.51*	1.16–1.95	9
Treatment location			
Prison	1.35*	1.16–1.56	27
Jail	1.56#	0.94–2.60	3
Length of treatment			
90 days or more	1.45*	1.26–1.68	22
Fewer than 90 days	1.15	0.79–1.67	3
Strictly voluntary treatment			
No	1.32*	1.08–1.61	8
Yes	1.57*	1.35–1.84	16
Program maturity			
New program (less than 1 year)	1.34*	1.10–1.64	14
Developing program (1–3 years)	1.18	0.79–1.77	4
Established program (3+ years)	1.45*	1.15–1.83	11

[a] Number of odds ratios
*$p<0.05$
#$p<0.10$

Note: From "Does incarceration-based drug treatment reduce recidivism? A meta-analytic synthesis of the research," by O.Mitchell, D.B. Wilson and D.L. MacKenzie, 2007, Journal of Experimental Criminology, 3(4), 353-375

Moreover the authors found that the programmes were slightly more effective in samples of females than in sample of either males or mixed sex. This finding was described by the authors as being food for thought given that it is known (see for instance, Pollock, 2004) that female inmates are much more likely to be drug abusers and that traditionally prison-based therapeutic communities are more easily accessible to males than females.

Four of the ten studies analysed by the authors also examined the impact of such programmes on drug relapse and generated mixed results. Of these four, two studies found that inmates who participated in prison therapeutic-community based programmes had lower rates of drug relapse when compared to those that did not, while the other two evaluations found the exact opposite. The overall mean odds ratio of these four studies was 1.02 (95% confidence interval 0.48 – 2.15) thus indicating no difference.

The existing evidence reviewed by Mitchell et al thus indicated that whilst prison therapeutic-community based programmes are associated with statistically significant decreases in recidivism, their impact, if any, on reducing drug relapse is less certain. The authors rightfully expressed their surprise at this finding since it has been traditionally assumed that the effectiveness of these programs in reducing recidivism is due to their success in reducing substance misuse. One would expect that the programmes would have the same impact on drug relapse as they have on recidivism or even possibly be more effective. Indeed, the study revealed a strong correlation between the odds ratios of drug relapse and the odds ratios of recidivism (unweighted 0.56, weighted 0.64) thus indicating that the more a program is effective on reducing drug relapse the more it is also effective on reducing recidivism.

The authors give two possible explanations for this unexpected finding of lower drug-relapse effects. The first is that using recidivism as a measure of effectiveness, itself a problematic notion and possible limiting factor, might be more reliable than using measures of drug relapse and that the latter are attenuated more than the former. The second possibility is that substance misuse may not mediate the relationship between such programs and criminal conduct and that while they may successfully be used to alter the criminogenic environment and the psycho-social issues that foster criminal conduct of inmates, they are unlikely to be as successful with regard to their drug use.

Mitchell et al. derived a number of other interesting conclusions from their meta-analytic study. They concluded that judicial authorities would do well to focus on intensive therapeutic community based programs for inmates that are incarcerated for drug-related offences. Conversely, the available evidence proved that smaller treatment benefits would ensure from programs that do not place emphasis on the multiple problems of such inmates and are less intensive.

They also established that there is not enough information and little or no studies dealing with the importance of specific components of therapeutic community based prison-inmate programs and whether reoffending rates may be influenced by the prevalence of one or more of such components or a combination of such components.

Finally the authors went to great length to emphasise on the fact that most of the evaluations analysed in their study were methodologically weak. In fact 20% of such evaluations were classified as weak quasi-experiments, 43% as standard quasi-experiments, 30% as rigorous quasi-experiments and 7% as experimental designs. There is therefore a possibility that being methodologically weak, the available research overestimates the effects of TC-based prison programmes on recidivism and there may be alternative explanations for reductions in recidivism other than due to the positive effects of the programmes.

In another study (Welsh, 2007), the author analysed the outcomes after release from prison over a period spanning 5 years post-release for 2,809 inmates who had participated in TC substance misuse treatment programs or control groups in a number of correctional facilities in Pennsylvania, US between January and November 2000. Data with regard to recidivism, rearrest and drug relapse for the experimental (TC) and control groups up to 5 years post-release was examined. Post-release data concerning reincarceration, rearrest, drug relapse and employment as well as pre-treatment data including demographics and criminal history was collected. It was found that participation in a TC-based program had a strongly significant effect on reducing recidivism over a five year post-release period ($p < .05$) and that this was independent of community aftercare. The impact on rearrest rates was slightly significant ($p < .09$) while that on drug relapse was negligible ($p > .10$). The author also found that with regard to two of the three analysed outcomes (i.e. recidivism and drug relapse), the severity of previous offences had no impact on recidivism and that employment after release from prison was the strongest predictor variable amongst all the outcomes. A recommendation was made to carry out further studies as to why in-prison drug treatment appears to be much more effective in reducing criminality than in drug-use.

Other studies were carried out to analyse the effectiveness of prison-TCs in Amity (California), Delaware and Texas. In California, the Amity prison TC has consistently been found to have a positive impact on those inmates who complete treatment (Prendergast, Hall, & Wexler, 2003; Wexler, De Leon, Thomas, Kressel & Peters, 1999). Wexler et al. (1999) found that program completers had substantially decreased rates of recidivism when compared to a no treatment comparison group at twelve and twenty-four months after release although this difference disappears at 36 months. Prendergast, Hall, Wexer, Melnick & Cao

(2004) however found that the significant reduction in recidivism persists even as late as five years after release.

A study on a therapeutic community in a Delaware prison that took into consideration outcomes after one year and a half established that program completers were less likely to relapse and demonstrated lower reconviction rates when compared to an untreated control group (Inciardi et al, 1997). A follow up study in 2004 concluded that participating in treatment was the single most important predictor of reoffending (Inciardi, Martin & Butzein, 2004).

Similar results were reported in Texas where Eisenberg and Fabelo (1996) found that after one year from release from prison, inmates who had been treated with a prison-based TC program exhibited lower rates of reconviction for a new offense or violation of parole than those who did not receive treatment or whose treatment had been discontinued.

Other studies reported a more marked difference in the outcomes on recidivism between those who attend and those who do not attend prison-based TCs. For instance, Hiller, Knight & Simpson (1999) found that inmates who completed the program in Kyle prison had a 50% less chance of recidivating than those that made up the comparison group.

The integration of CBT treatment with TC-based programmes has been found to a very effective drug treatment approach in prison settings (Malinowski, 2003). It is based on the premise that offenders have different ways of thinking, lack suitable social skills, and generally operate from a lower level of moral development (Prendergast et al., 2004). The aim of CBT is to help inmates alter their thought processes to correct dysfunctional and criminogenic thinking patterns (Landenberger & Lipsey, 2005).

Pelissier, Motivans & Rounds Bryant (2005) analysed twenty federal prison programmes that incorporated CBT and found positive outcomes for recidivism and drug use in sixteen programmes.

Miller (2010) conducted a quasi-experimental post-test only retrospective study using data obtained through the Department of Public Safety and Correctional Services in Maryland, US to analyse the relationship between in-prison substance treatment for female inmates as well as severity of addiction on rates of recidivism. Treatment consisted of either a therapeutic community program or a six-month outpatient CBT program. The study included three groups of female inmates with a past history of drug dependence that were released from Maryland Correctional Institution for Women: one group consisted of inmates who had competed the TC program before release, another group consisted of inmates who had completed the CBT program and the comparison group consisted of such inmates that did not receive any substance abuse treatment prior to release.

The first part of the study analysed the hypothesis that inmates who completed any form of treatment (i.e. whether TC-based program or CBT program) before release would be less likely to recidivate than those who did not. Logistic regression analysis for the hypothesis was carried out and it turned out to be non-significant. The predictor variables that were included in the analysis simultaneously were treatment (whether TC-based or CBT based), race, age, number of previous incarcerations and number of years after release). The Wald chi-square for the coefficient associated with treatment was statistically insignificant, $\chi^2(1) = 1.28, p = .258$ thus meaning that participation in prison-based substance abuse treatment was not found to be a significant predictor of recidivism. An interesting finding that did emerge was that the likelihood of recidivism was almost one and a half times more for each additional prior incarceration ($p = .002$).

31

The second part of the study analysed the hypothesis that inmates who participated in the TC-based program before release would be less likely to recidivate than those that participated in the CBT-based program. The same predictor variables were included simultaneously in the logical regression analysis. The result of this analysis for such hypothesis was also insignificant. The Wald chi-square for the coefficient associated with the TC-based group was $\chi^2(1) = .247$, $p = .619$ thus meaning that completion of the TC was not a significant predictor of recidivism compared to the CBT-based group. None of the other predictor variables reached significance.

The third part of the study analysed the hypothesis that inmates with a higher severity of addiction would be more likely to recidivate than those with a less severity of addiction. Logistic regression was carried out to determine whether severity of addiction is a significant predictor of recidivism. Severity of addiction was measured using the Addiction Severity Index (ASI) ratings ranging from 4 (low) to 9 (high). The same predictor variables were included simultaneously in the logical regression analysis. The Wald chi-square for the coefficient associated with severity of addiction was statistically insignificant, $\chi^2(1) = .001$, $p = .974$ thus meaning that severity of addiction was not found to be a significant predictor of recidivism. In this study, treatment and severity of addiction were not determined to be significant predictors of recidivism. However reincarceration was still higher among those who did not complete treatment prior to release from prison than those who did. Notwithstanding the lack of statistical significance, the author concluded that the practical importance of providing prison-based substance abuse treatment should not be dismissed.

Other possible predictors of recidivism

The literature review makes a strong case for the existence of such other predictor variables that have a significant effect on reducing reincarceration. As already highlighted, in testing the hypothesis that participation in prison-based substance abuse treatment is a significant predictor of recidivism, Miller (2010) found that the likelihood of recidivism was almost one and a half times more for each additional prior incarceration ($p = .002$). Also, Welsh (2007) reported that post-release employment was the strongest predictor variable (out of various other predictors analysed in his study) of the outcomes of reincarceration, rearrest and drug relapse.

The number of prior arrests has also been found to be a significant predictor of recidivism (Inciardi et al., 2004, Welsh, 2007; Wexler et al., 1999). Also, offenders who are employed and have stable housing are reported to have a lower risk of recidivating (Messina, Burdon, Hagopian & Prendergast, 2006). With regard to psychological status, it has been reported that inmates with co-existing disorders were more likely to recidivate (Messina et al., 2006.) as were those whose drug problem was more severe or whose drug of choice was heroin (Gossop et al., 2005).

Another interesting significant predictor of recidivism is sex. Inciardi et al. (2004) found that it is significantly less likely for a female inmate who undertakes prison-based treatment to recidivate than a male inmate. Messina et al. (2006) shared this finding when they attempted to examine the influence of gender on recidivism rates. They reported that male recidivists were reconvicted significantly sooner than their female counterparts. Furthermore, they found that a number of predictor variables demonstrated different effects on recidivism between sexes. For instance, one's race and employment status before incarceration was a predictor of recidivism for males but not for females, while the total time

33

spent in substance use treatment and one's education background prior to incarceration were strong predictors for females but not for males. However co-existing disorders and total period of incarceration in one's lifetime were significant recidivism predictors in both sexes.

It has also been reported that retention is a significant predictor of long-term success and that the effects of participation in TC-based programs on recidivism are most consistent for treatment completers rather than for dropouts (De Leon, 2000).

Conclusion

The research evidence clearly proves that substance abuse treatment that is based on TC is effective in reducing rates of recidivism for substance involved offenders. The positive outcomes associated with providing such treatment to inmates translates into decreased criminal conduct, possibly reduced incidence of drug use, safer prison environments and cost savings that ultimately benefit society at large.

Chapter 4: Data Collection and Analysis

The purpose of this study was to examine the relationship between in-prison drug rehabilitation programmes for inmates at the Corradino Correctional Facility and recidivism. The study assessed retrospectively whether recidivism among substance dependent inmates was less likely for offenders who participated in such program prior to their release. Additionally the study examined the relationship between completion of drug rehabilitation programmes (as against participating and dropping out) and recidivism.

Data Collection

The present study is a quasi-experimental retrospective cohort study designed to determine the impact of prison inmate programmes on recidivism amongst inmates at the Corradino Correctional Facility. Existing data consisting in electronic files maintained and kept at the Corradino Correctional Facility by dedicated individuals was collected. These files contained extensive information on inmates admitted to the Corradino Correctional Facility since 1946 including date of birth, age at admission, occupational status, type of conviction and date of sentences. Other files contained information with regard to participation in prison inmate programmes, psychiatric treatment pre-admission, psychiatric treatment post-admission and substance-replacement therapy in the Corradino Correctional Facility. The latter files were compiled on inmates admitted to the Corradino Correctional Facility in the last decade or so.

Data was gathered on three groups of inmates having a history of substance abuse all of whom were released from the Corradino Correctional Facility between 2005 and 2008. The total sample size for use in this study consisted of 361 inmates. The sample size for the first analysis in the present study included 361 inmates while that for the second analysis was delimited to 105 inmates.

Research Question Number One

The first research question examined whether offenders with substance disorder who participated in a prison inmate program would be less likely to reoffend than offenders who did not take part in any such program. For this analysis, the following three groups were compared, that is, the group (coded 1) consisting of all inmates who did not participate in any prison-inmate programme during the time spent in prison for a conviction that ended between 2005 and 2008 but who had participated in a prison-inmate programme in the past (n=27), the group (coded 2) consisting of all inmates who were released from the Corradino Correctional Facility between 2005 and 2008 and who never participated in any prison inmate programme (n=229) and the group (coded 3) consisting of all inmates who participated in at least one of the prison inmate programmes during the time spent in prison for a conviction that ended between 2005 and 2008 (n=105).

The covariate predictors of sex, age on admission, age of first conviction, occupation, in-prison psychiatric treatment, in-prison drug replacement treatment and number of prior incarcerations were included in the analysis since these could possibly be predictive of the outcome under study as evidenced in the literature review. Other factors found to predict recidivism in the literature review such as social support, educational level, participation in aftercare and duration of post-release period from prison were not available for inclusion in the analysis.

36

It was hypothesized that participation in a prison-inmate program would result in lower recidivism than for those drug offenders who did not participate in such programmes prior to release from prison or who had participated in the past.

Statistical Analysis

PASW Statistics (formerly SPSS) version 18.0.0 was used for data analysis. Pearson chi-square tests, Fisher's Exact Test and a Generalised Linear Model with a logit link function were used to compare categorical variables (including sex, occupation, in-prison replacement treatment, in-prison psychiatric treatment and the number of previous convictions) between groups, ascertain any possible relationship between recidivism and such variables and ultimately test the null hypothesis. The variable "number of previous convictions" was included as a categorical variable coded as follows: 0 = no previous convictions, 1 = one previous conviction, 2 = two previous convictions and 3 = three or more previous convictions.

For the continuous variable of age on admission a one way analysis of variance (ANOVA) was used. An alpha level of .05 for all statistical tests was used.

Descriptive Data

The variable of sex was coded as 1 = male, 2 = female. In Group 1 (those inmates who had attended a prison-inmate program in the past but not during the time spent in prison for a conviction that ended between 2005 and 2008) 27 inmates (100%) were males and none (0%) were females, in Group 2 (those inmates who never participated in any prison inmate programme) 213 inmates (93%) were males and 16 (7%) were females, whilst in Group 3 (those inmates who participated in a prison inmate program during the time spent in prison for a conviction that ended between 2005 and 2008) 98 inmates (93%) were males and 7 (7%) were females. A crosstab of study participants by sex is shown in Appendix A (Table A1).

Age on admission ranged from 14 to 59 years of age with a mean age of 29.15 ($SD =$ 8.47). The mean age on admission for Group 1 was 29.85 years ($SD = 5.88$), for Group 2 was 29.5 years ($SD = 9.15$) and for Group 3 was 28.21 years ($SD = 7.4$). Table A2 in Appendix A shows some descriptive statistics of the study participants by age on admission.

Age at first conviction also ranged from 14 to 59 years of age with a mean age of 26.31 ($SD = 7.33$). The mean age at first conviction for Group 1 was 25.11 years ($SD = 5.15$), for Group 2 was 27.31 years ($SD = 7.96$) and for Group 3 was 24.46 years ($SD = 5.85$). Table A3 in Appendix A shows some descriptive statistics of the study participants by age at first conviction.

The variable "occupation" was included as a dichotomous categorical variable coded as follows: 0=unemployed on admission, 1=employed on admission. In Group 1, 26 (96%) inmates were unemployed and one (4%) inmate was employed. In Group 2, 177 (77%) inmates were unemployed and 52 (33%) inmates were employed. In Group 3, 82 (78%) inmates were unemployed and 23 (22%) inmates were employed. A crosstab of study participants by occupation is shown in Appendix A in Table A4.

Table 2 presents a summary of the descriptive data for the study participants with regard to sex, age on admission, age at first conviction and occupation.

Table 2

Summary of descriptive data in relation to sex, age on admission, age at first conviction and occupation

Variable	Group 1 (*n* = 27)	Group 2 (*n* = 229)	Group 3 (*n* = 105)	Total (N = 361)
Sex # Males (%)	27 (100)	213 (93)	98 (93)	338 (94)
Sex # Females (%)	0 (0)	16 (7)	7 (7)	23 (6)
Mean age on admission (SD)	29.85 (5.88)	29.5 (9.15)	28.21 (7.4)	29.15 (8.47)
Mean age on 1st conviction (SD)	25.11 (5.15)	27.31 (7.96)	24.46 (5.85)	26.31 (7.33)
Occupation # Unemployed (%)	26 (96)	177 (77)	82 (78)	285 (79)
Occupation # Employed (%)	1 (4)	52 (33)	23 (22)	76 (21)

Notes: *Group 1 - inmates who attended PiP in the past, Group 2 - inmates who never participated in PiP, Group 3 - inmates who participated in a PiP in reference period*

Table A5 in Appendix A presents a crosstab of recidivism for participants in the three groups. The outcome variable of recidivism was coded as 1=yes and 0=no. Forty-eight percent of all study participants reoffended. Recidivism was found in 70 % of Group 1, 42.4% of Group 2, and 55% of Group 3.

Offences were classified in terms of the main titles of the Criminal Code, i.e. offences against property (including theft, fraud and misappropriation), offences against the person (including grievous bodily harm, homicide and sexual offences), conversion of administrative fines (i.e. conversion of unpaid court experts fees and unpaid court-imposed fines into custodial sentences), breach of court-imposed conditions (i.e. breach of bail or probation), drug offences and other offences (including perjury and corruption). As can be seen by the frequencies cross tabulated in Appendix A (Table A6), with regard to the profile of offences on admission, in Groups 1 and 3, the most common offences were those against property followed by drug offences whilst in Group 2, the most common were drug offences followed by crimes against property. Conversion of administrative fines into custodial sentences was particularly higher in Group 2. Conversely, in Group 3 the least common offences were conversion of administrative fines into custodial sentences and breach of court-imposed conditions.

As can be seen by the frequencies cross tabulated in Appendix A (Table A7), with regard to the profile of re-offences, in all groups the most common offences for which inmates were convicted after release from prison were offences against property. Interestingly, in Groups 2 and 3 the second most common re-offences consisted in conversion of administrative fines into custodial sentences.

The variable "number of previous convictions" was included as a categorical variable coded as follows: 0 = no previous convictions, 1 = one previous conviction, 2 = two previous convictions and 3+ = three or more previous convictions. Group 2 had the highest number of no previous convictions as demonstrated in Appendix A (Table A8).

The variable of in-prison replacement treatment was coded as 0=no replacement treatment, 1=on tramadol only, 2=on methadone treatment with or without tramadol. In Group 1, 74% were on methadone, 7% on tramadol only and only 18% were not administered any replacement treatment. In Group 2, 52% were on methadone, 11% were on tramadol only and 37% were on no replacement treatment. No replacement treatment was most common in Group 2. In Group 3, 74% were on methadone, 10% were on tramadol only and 16% were on no replacement treatment. A crosstab of study participants by in-prison replacement treatment is shown in Appendix A (Table A9).

The variable of in-prison psychiatric treatment was coded as 0=no psychiatric treatment, 1=on psychiatric treatment. Inmates in Group 2 were the least likely to be on psychiatric treatment. In Groups 1 and 3, 89% were on psychiatric treatment, whilst in Group 2 this was 69%. A crosstab of study participants by psychiatric replacement treatment is shown in Appendix A (Table A10).

Results

There was no statistically significant difference between groups with regard to sex, $p = .537$ (2-tailed). For this analysis a Fisher's Exact Test (Appendix A, Table A11) was used since once cell had an expected count of less than 1. There was also no difference between the percentage of females in the total sample and the percentage of females participating in one of the prison inmate programs.

There was also no statistically significant difference between groups with regard to age on admission, $F (2, 358) = 9.38$, p=.392, and occupation, $\chi^2 (2, N = 361) = 5.31$, $p = .070$. Tables A12 and A13 in Appendix A show the ANOVA and chi-square tests used for these analyses.

There was a highly significant difference between groups with regard to the number of previous convictions $\chi^2(6, N = 361) = 32.51$, $p < .001$, the variable of in-prison replacement treatment $\chi^2(4, N = 361) = 18.44$, $p = .001$, and the variable of in-prison psychiatric treatment $\chi^2(2, N = 361) = 18.69$, $p < .001$. The chi-square tests used in these analyses are shown in Appendix A (Tables A14, A15 and A16 respectively).

41

Collinearity was observed between replacement treatment and psychiatric treatment. In fact 89% of inmates who were administered replacement treatment were also on psychiatric treatment, whilst only 46% of those who were not having replacement treatment were on psychiatric treatment. It was thus decided that psychiatric treatment should be eliminated from further statistical analysis.

With regard to recidivism rates an initial chi-squared analysis revealed a highly significant difference between groups $\chi^2(2, N = 361) = 10.53, p = .005$, as shown in Appendix A (Table A17). A generalized linear model with a logit link function was thus used to compare the reoffence rate between groups when controlling for replacement treatment and the number of previous convictions. This is shown in Table 3. It emerged that the difference between groups was not significant when controlling for replacement treatment and number of previous convictions and thus the null hypothesis was not rejected. It was found that those inmates who were not administered any replacement treatment were 74% less likely to reoffend compared to those who were given methadone or tramadol. Interestingly, the number of previous convictions emerged as a significant predictor of recidivism. Results indicated that the likelihood of recidivism was 1.7 times greater for each additional prior incarceration (p < .001).

Table 3

Parameter Estimates - Comparison of reoffence rate between groups when controlling for replacement treatment and number of previous convictions

Parameter	B	Std. Error	95% Wald Confidence Interval		Hypothesis Test				95% Wald Confidence Interval for Exp(B)	
			Lower	Upper	Wald Chi-Square	df	Sig.	Exp(B)	Lower	Upper
Group = 1	.665	.4985	-.312	1.642	1.781	1	.182	1.945	.732	5.167
Group = 2	-.088	.2638	-.605	.429	.112	1	.738	.915	.546	1.535
Group = 3	.	.	.	.	.	.	.	1	.	.
PREV[c]	.571	.1177	.341	.802	23.561	1	.000	1.770	1.406	2.230
[REPL=0][d]	-1.329	.2829	-1.883	-.774	22.061	1	.000	.265	.152	.461
[REPL=1][e]	.159	.3773	-.581	.898	.177	1	.674	1.172	.559	2.455
[REPL=2][f]	1[b]	.	.	.	.	.	.	1	.	.

Dependent Variable: Reoffending

Model: (Intercept), Group, PREV, REPL

a. Set to zero because this parameter is redundant.

b. Fixed at the displayed value.

c. Number of previous convictions

d. No in-prison replacement treatment

e. In-prison replacement treatment - on tramadol only

f. In-prison replacement treatment - on methadone treatment with or without tramadol

Research Question Number Two

The second research question examined whether offenders with substance disorder who completed the prison inmate programme would be less likely to reoffend than offenders who did not complete the programme. For this analysis, the group (formerly coded 3) consisting of all inmates who participated in at least one of the prison inmate programmes during the time spent in prison for a conviction that ended between 2005 and 2008 (n=105) was split into two groups. One group (coded 1) consisted of those who had completed the prison inmate program (n=48) while the other group (coded 2) consisted of those who had dropped out of such program (n=57).

The covariate predictors of sex, program type, age on admission, age of first conviction, occupation, in-prison psychiatric treatment, in-prison drug replacement treatment and number of prior incarcerations were included in the analysis since these could possibly be predictive of the outcome under study as evidenced in the literature review. Other factors found to predict recidivism in the literature review such as social support, educational level, participation in aftercare and duration of post-release period from prison were not available for inclusion in the analysis.

It was hypothesized that completion of a prison-inmate program would result in lower recidivism rates when compared to those drug offenders who dropped out from any such program.

Statistical Analysis

PASW Statistics (formerly SPSS) version 18.0.0 was used for data analysis. Pearson chi-square tests, Fisher's Exact Test and a Generalised Linear Model with a logit link function were used to compare categorical variables (including sex, occupation, in-prison

44

replacement treatment, in-prison psychiatric treatment, the number of previous convictions and type of program) between groups, ascertain any possible relationship between recidivism and such variables and ultimately test the null hypothesis. The variable "number of previous convictions" was included as a categorical variable coded as follows: 0 = no previous convictions, 1 = one previous conviction, 2 = two previous convictions and 3 = three or more previous convictions.

For the continuous variables of age on admission and age on first conviction independent t-tests were used. An alpha level of .05 for all statistical tests was used.

Descriptive Data

The variable of sex was coded as 1 = male, 2 = female. In Group 1 (completers) 48 inmates (100%) were males and none were females whilst in Group 2 (dropouts) 50 inmates (88%) were males and 7 (12%) were females. A crosstab of study participants by sex is shown in Appendix B (Table B1).

Age on admission ranged from 16 to 50 years of age with a mean age of 28.21 (SD = 7.40). The mean age on admission for Group 1 was 28.92 years (SD = 7.04) whilst that for Group 2 was 27.61 years (SD = 7.69).

Age at first conviction ranged from 15 to 41 years of age with a mean age of 24.46 (SD = 5.85). The mean age at first conviction for Group 1 was 25.23 years (SD = 5.69) whilst that for Group 2 was 23.81 years (SD = 5.96). Tables B2 and B3 in Appendix B show some descriptive statistics of the study participants by age on admission and age at first conviction.

The variable "occupation" was included as a dichotomous categorical variable coded as follows: 0=unemployed on admission, 1=employed on admission. In Group 1, 32 (67%) inmates were unemployed and sixteen inmates were employed (33%) whilst in Group 2, 50

(88%) inmates were unemployed and 7 (12%) inmates were employed. A crosstab of study participants by occupation is shown in Table B4 in Appendix B.

Table 4 presents a summary of the descriptive data for the study participants with regard to sex, age on admission, age at first conviction and occupation.

Table 4

Summary of descriptive data in relation to sex, age on admission, age at first conviction and occupation

Variable	Group 1 (*n* = 48)	Group 2 (*n* = 57)	Total (N = 105)
Sex # Males (%)	48 (100)	50 (88)	98(93)
Sex # Females (%)	0 (0)	7 (12)	7 (7)
Mean age on admission (SD)	28.92 (7.04)	27.61 (7.70)	28.21 (7.40)
Mean age on 1st conviction (SD)	25.23 (5.69)	23.81 (5.96)	24.46 (5.85)
Occupation # Unemployed (%)	32 (67)	50 (88)	82 (78)
Occupation # Employed (%)	16 (33)	7(12)	23 (22)

Notes: *Group 1 - inmates who attended and completed PiP in the past, Group 2 - inmates who attended but dropped out from a PiP*

Table B5 in Appendix B presents a crosstab of recidivism for participants in the two groups. The outcome variable of recidivism was coded as 1=yes and 0=no. 55% of all study participants reoffended. Recidivism was found in 45.8 % of Group 1 and 63.2% of Group 2.

Offences were classified in terms of the main titles of the Criminal Code, i.e. offences against property (including theft, fraud and misappropriation), offences against the person (including grievous bodily harm, homicide and sexual offences), conversion of administrative fines (i.e. conversion of unpaid court experts fees and unpaid court-imposed fines into custodial sentences), breach of court-imposed conditions (i.e. breach of bail or probation), drug offences and other offences (including perjury and corruption). As can be seen by the frequencies cross tabulated in Appendix B (Table B6), with regard to the profile of offences on admission, in both groups, the most common offences were those against property followed by drug offences.

As can also be seen by the frequencies cross tabulated in Appendix B (Table B7), with regard to the profile of re-offences, in Group 1, the most common offences for which inmates were convicted after release from prison were offences against property (73%) followed by conversion of administrative fines into custodial sentences (27%) whilst in Group 2 the most common re-offences were offences against property (58%) followed by drug offences (14%). Interestingly, in Group 1 (i.e. those inmates who completed the program) no inmate re-entered prison on a drug offence.

The prison inmate programmes were coded as follows, SATU=1, SEDQA=2 and CARITAS=3. Those who participated in the prison inmate program operated by Sedqa performed slightly better with regards to recidivism than those who participated in the other programs as evidenced by the crosstab in Appendix B (Table B8).

The variable "number of previous convictions" was included as a categorical variable coded as follows: 0 = no previous convictions, 1 = one previous conviction, 2 = two previous convictions and 3+ = three or more previous convictions. In both Group 1 (60.4%) and Group 2 (43.9%) the majority of inmates had no previous convictions as demonstrated in Appendix B (Table B9).

The variable of in-prison replacement treatment was coded as 0=no replacement treatment, 1=on tramadol only, 2=on methadone treatment with or without tramadol. In both Group 1 (88%) and Group 2 (90%) the absolute majority of inmates were on methadone treatment with or without tramadol. A crosstab of study participants by in-prison replacement treatment is shown in Appendix B (Table B10).

48

The variable of in-prison psychiatric treatment was coded as 0=no psychiatric treatment, 1=on psychiatric treatment. In Group 1, 80 % were on psychiatric treatment and 21% were not, whilst in Group 2, 99% were on psychiatric treatment and only 2% were not. A crosstab of study participants by in-prison replacement treatment is shown in Appendix B (Table B11).

Results

There was a statistically significant difference between groups with regard to sex, $p = .015$ (2-tailed) and occupation, $\chi^2(1, N = 105) = 6.75, p = .009$, as shown in Appendix B (Tables B12 and B13 respectively).

There was no significant difference between groups with regard to age on admission, $t(103) = .90$, p =.371, age at first conviction, $t(103) = 1.24$, p =.216, the number of previous convictions, $\chi^2(3, N = 105) = 3.66, p = .300$ and the variable of in-prison replacement treatment, $\chi^2(2, N = 105) = .548, p = .760$ as shown in Appendix B (Tables B14, B15, B16 and B17 respectively).

There was however a highly significant difference between groups with regard to in-prison psychiatric treatment, $\chi^2(1, N = 105) = 10.11, p = .001$ as shown in Appendix B (Table B18).

While those who participated in the prison inmate program operated by Sedqa performed slightly better with regards to recidivism than those who participated in the other programs, this difference does not achieve significance, $\chi^2(2, N = 105) = .959, p = .619$ as demonstrated in Appendix B (Table B18).

49

With regard to recidivism rates between groups, there was a difference in that whilst in Group 1 (completers), 46% % reoffended and 55% did not, in Group 2 (drop outs), 63% reoffended and 37% did not. A chi-square analysis (shown in Appendix B Table B19) however demonstrated that, while close, this difference did not achieve statistical significance, $\chi^2(1, N = 105) = 3.16, p = .075$ though it might well reach significance with a larger sample size. When adjusting for sex, occupation and in-prison psychiatric treatment (by using a generalized linear model with a logit link function) the difference between groups became clearly insignificant and thus the null hypothesis was not rejected. This is shown in Table 5. It was also found that males were almost six times more likely to recidivate than females, that being on psychiatric treatment increases the risk of recidivating by five and a half times and that being unemployed on admission increases such risk by more than one and a half time.

Table 5

Parameter Estimates - Comparison of reoffence rate between groups when controlling for occupation, in-prison psychiatric treatment and sex

Parameter	B	Std. Error	95% Wald Confidence Interval		Hypothesis Test				95% Wald Confidence Interval for Exp(B)	
			Lower	Upper	Wald Chi-Square	df	Sig.	Exp(B)	Lower	Upper
Group 1	-.565	.4533	-1.453	.324	1.551	1	.213	.569	.234	1.383
Group 2	.	.	.	.	.	.	.	1	.	.
[OCC=0]c	.499	.5160	-.513	1.510	.934	1	.334	1.646	.599	4.527
[OCC=1]d	.	.	.	.	.	.	.	1	.	.
PSYe	1.689	.8375	.048	3.331	4.069	1	.044	5.416	1.049	27.961
[SEX=1]f	1.780	.8949	.026	3.534	3.957	1	.047	5.930	1.026	34.261
[SEX=2]g	1b	.	.	.	.	.	.	1	.	.

Dependent Variable: REOFF

Model: (Intercept), GRP, OCC, PSY, SEX

a. Set to zero because this parameter is redundant.
b. Fixed at the displayed value.
c. Unemployed on admission
d. Employed on admission
e. In-prison psychiatric treatment
f. Males
g. Females

51

Chapter 5: Conclusions and Recommendations

Major Findings

In this study it was hypothesized that recidivism would be significantly reduced for inmates who participated in prison inmate programs and that those who actually completed a program were less likely to reoffend than those who did not.

With regard to the first hypothesis, a generalized linear model with a logit link function was employed and it was established that the difference between groups was not significant when controlling for replacement treatment and the number of previous convictions and thus the null hypothesis was not rejected. Indeed, quite surprisingly recidivism was higher in the treatment group (55.2%) than in the group who never participated in a program. Thus in-prison substance abuse treatment was not a significant predictor of recidivism for inmates at the Corradino Correctional Facility in this study.

In keeping with findings from other studies (Gossop et al., 2005) that reported that inmates whose drug problem was more severe were more likely to recidivate, it was found that those inmates who were not administered any drug replacement treatment were 74% less likely to reoffend compared to those who were given methadone or tramadol.

Also, the finding that the likelihood of recidivism was 1.7 times greater for each additional prior incarceration (p < .001) replicated the findings of earlier studies (Hiller et al., 1999; Martin et al, 1999; Mosher et al., 2006) that reported that the number of previous convictions is a significant predictor of recidivism.

Age on admission ($p = .392$) was found not to be a significant predictor of recidivism despite the consistent finding reported in other studies (Gossop et al., 2005, Inciardi et al.,

52

2004, Messin et al., 20006 and Welsh, 2007) that younger offenders were most likely to recidivate.

With regard to the second hypothesis, a generalized linear model with a logit link function was also employed and it was established that the difference between groups was not significant when controlling for sex, occupation and in-prison psychiatric treatment and thus the null hypothesis was not rejected. Thus completion of prison-based substance abuse treatment (as against mere participation) was not a significant predictor of recidivism for inmates at the Corradino Correctional Facility in this study. Despite this lack of statistical significance it must however be noted that recidivism was higher for drop-outs (63%) than for completers (46%). Therefore the possibility that completing a prison inmate program leads to lower recidivism cannot be dismissed outright irrespective of the finding of the statistical insignificance. Indeed, a larger sample might have led to a finding of significance.

It was found that males are almost six times more likely to reoffend than females although this finding needs to be interpreted with caution given the very low number of females who participated in prison inmate programs. In this regard mention must be made of the finding that there was no difference between the percentage of females in the total sample (6.3%) and the percentage of females participating in one of the prison inmate programs (6.6%) thus indicating that such programs are equally accessible to both sexes. Also, it was established that being unemployed upon admission increased the risk of reoffending by more than one and a half times. Both these findings concur with previous studies that reported that gender and employment status are significant predictors of recidivism (Inciardi et al., 2004, Welsh, 2007).

An important finding was that those who were on psychiatric treatment were 5.5 times more likely of recidivating than those who were not. This accords with other studies that

53

reported that inmates with co-existing disorders were more likely to reoffend (Messina et. al., 2006).

The study also determined that there was no significant difference in recidivism rates between the three prison inmate programs (p = .619) although Sedqa (48.6% recidivism rate) fared slightly better when compared with SATU (59.4%) and CARITAS (57.9%). There was also no significant difference in retention rates between the three programs (p = .916).

Limitations

Acknowledging the possible limitations of a study is important not only due to the possibility of such limitations having influenced the results but also since it is an opportunity to put forward suggestions for additional research.

Primarily, being of a quasi-experimental design, this study studies pre-established groups of subjects rather than subjects that have been randomly assigned to experimental conditions, that is, participants are not randomly assigned to levels of the independent variable (i.e. recidivism).

This type of design was appropriate and indeed made necessary because the researcher used existing archived data (consisting in electronic files maintained and kept at the Corradino Correctional Facility) and thus it was neither possible nor feasible to randomly assign individuals to groups.

The main problem with a quasi-experimental retrospective design (as against a true experimental design) is that there is a real risk that results could be due to one or more confounding variables. Quasi-experiments tend to have lower internal validity in comparison to true experiments and it may be difficult to interpret results as group equivalence is not assumed. In this study, the analysis included two comparison groups to help control for some

54

of the variance. This notwithstanding, selection bias remains a real threat to the internal validity of this study. A number of covariate predictor variables that were available to include in the analysis some of whom were identified in the literature review (including age on admission, number of prior incarcerations, in-prison psychiatric treatment, in-prison replacement treatment and occupational status) were entered so as to adjust for possible differences between the groups on available variables. However other factors found to predict recidivism in the literature review such as social support, educational level, participation in aftercare and duration of post-release period from prison were not available for inclusion in the analysis.

Secondly, being of a retrospective design, the researcher did not have control on the choice, accuracy or completeness of the data presented to her. Almost all data consisted in archived electronic files painstakingly compiled, maintained and kept at the Corradino Correctional Facility by dedicated individuals who were neither trained nor paid for carrying out such an important task. Yet the researcher cannot vouch for the completeness of the data and there are no guarantees whatsoever that all information had been inputted in an accurate manner and as expected. The limitation of the design of the study also meant that the author could not control for variables that were missing from the data and which have been reported as being significant predictors of recidivism in other studies. For instance data regarding possible confounding variables after release from prison was not available and since the research design did not include personal contact with subjects to evaluate post-release activities and living conditions such data could not be collected. Factors such as social support, living environment, employment status and participation in aftercare post-release from prison have all been found to be strongly linked with recidivism (Welsh, 2007, Hepburn, 2005). Data concerning drug relapse after release from prison would also have been useful in view of a number of studies that determined that the more a prison-inmate program is effective on reducing drug relapse the more it is also effective on reducing recidivism. The lack of access to prisoners also meant that carrying out face-to-face interviews to measure and control for inmates' characteristics (including motivation), programmatic variations and environments, all of which have been identified as predictors of recidivism (Wexler et al., 1999), was not possible.

Thirdly, using recidivism as an outcome measure has a number of possible limitations. For the purpose of this study, recidivism was defined as a conviction by the Maltese Courts, occurring after release from prison between 2005 and 2008, necessitating a custodial sentence and re-entry into prison. Therefore an inmate who was released between 2005 and 2008, reoffended, was convicted by Court but was awarded a non-custodial sentence (such as a suspended sentence) was not considered a recidivist for the purpose of this study. On the other hand, an inmate who was released between 2005 and 2008, did not reoffend but was convicted by Court and awarded a custodial sentence for a crime that was committed in the past was considered a recidivist. This means that recidivism rates at least within the scope of this study may be inaccurate and/or misleading since a decrease or increase in such rates might not necessarily reflect a genuine decrease or increase in reoffending but might reflect unrelated factors such as commission of less detectable offences, or more likely, delays in the processing and conviction of offenders for pending charges (unfortunately a common occurrence in the local justice system). These factors must therefore be considered as limiting factors since they might influence the reliability of recidivism as an outcome variable. Furthermore, recidivism rates may be influenced by factors (including psycho-social circumstances and environmental considerations) that are independent of the participation or otherwise in a prison inmate program.

It must also be pointed out that using recidivism in general as a performance indicator does not take into consideration the seriousness of the crime for which an inmate is reincarcerated. For instance, in the analysis for hypothesis one, more than 23% of reoffenders were reincarcerated for administrative penalties consisting, more often than not, in failure by inmates to pay fines or fees in relation to previous criminal cases for which they had been incarcerated. This contrasts with the significantly lesser percentage of reoffenders (i.e. almost 13%) that were reconvicted for drug-related offences.

The period over which recidivism is measured will also inevitably influence the extent of recidivism that is uncovered. In this study recidivism was measured over the period spanning from the release date (any day between 1st January 2005 and 31st December 2008) till the end of 2012. One reasonably expects that the longer the period of time taken into consideration the higher the rate of recidivism that might be uncovered. For instance, Wexler et al. (1999) established that inmates who completed a prison Therapeutic Community program in Amity, California, had significantly lower rates of recidivism than a no treatment control group at twelve and twenty-four months after release but this difference disappeared at 36 months. Therefore a shorter follow up period in this study would have possibly led to different results. Conversely, a longer follow-up period might have possibly led to a decrease in the difference (already statistically insignificant) in recidivism rates between groups.

Also, putting emphasis on recidivism as an outcome variable to measure performance of prison-inmate programmes might render other equally important variables (such as the health, education, psychological or employment status of inmates post release) redundant. It is possible that the success of participation in a prison-inmate program is better measured by means of an assessment of such other variables.

Another possible limitation of this study is the sample size. While the sample sizes in the present study (361 inmates for the first analysis and 105 inmates for the second analysis) were deemed modest but adequate for the proposed study design, the possibility that larger samples might have led to significant differences in recidivism rates cannot be discounted. Indeed studies identified in the literature review that reported significant treatment effects utilised larger samples ranging from 690 (Inciardi et al., 2004) to 715 (Prendergast et al., 2004) and 1,343 inmates (Pelissier et al., 2005).

Conclusion

The present study failed to replicate the findings of a large number of studies, most of which conducted in the United States, that participation in-prison substance abuse treatment based on the therapeutic community model is a significant predictor of recidivism. While the limitations of the study, especially the study design and modest sample size, are important considerations when evaluating its outcomes, a possibility that cannot be excluded is that the prison inmate programs offered to inmates at the Corradino Correctional Facility are not accomplishing their intended objectives and goals at least in terms of ensuring that clients do not return to prison. On the other hand, lack of supervision, support and community after care post-release from the programs might be defining factors that influence and possibly eliminate the possible benefits ensuing to inmates from participation.

Future research should ideally be conducted using a large sample and a different design, perhaps incorporating a longitudinal perspective that includes face to face interviews with inmates and analyses of the influence on treatment outcomes of factors such as variations between the programs, the duration of such programs, inmates' characteristics,

58

post-release psycho-social stressors and confounding variables such as social support, employment status and participation in aftercare.

This study also found that inmates who were not given drug replacement treatment during their stay in prison (thus indicating that their drug problem was less severe) were 74% less likely to reoffend compared to those who were and that repeat offenders were at a higher risk of reoffending (the likelihood of recidivism was 1.7 times greater for each additional prior incarceration). Within the group of program participants, it was found that recidivism was higher for drop-outs (63%) than for completers (46%) although the difference did not achieve significance, that males are almost six times more likely to reoffend than females, that being unemployed upon admission increased the risk of reoffending by more than 1.5 times and that those on psychiatric treatment were 5.5 times more likely to recidivate than those who were not. All these findings need to be interpreted with caution given the stated limitations. At the same time attention to such factors that have been associated with recidivism in this study would be warranted in future evaluations of the prison inmate programs. It would for instance appear prudent to place greater emphasis on the psychiatric well-being of participants with co-existing disorders perhaps by varying the structure of the programs to give more importance and emphasis on psychiatric aspects, through the assistance of psychiatrists. The problem of retention also needs to be addressed. The effect of not completing a program on recidivism was close to significance in this study and might indeed have reached significance with a larger sample. While it is understandable that clients that do not obey the rules or do not follow the expected progress are dismissed it might be worth considering other forms of sanctions short of termination from participation in such programs.

A significant finding reported in the first hypothesis of this study was that more than 23% of reoffenders were reincarcerated for administrative penalties consisting in failure to pay fines or fees in relation to previous criminal cases. It would appear harsh and counter-productive for an inmate who having diligently followed and completed a prison inmate program is released with optimistic hopes for a better future only to be sent back to prison for failing to pay such fines. It would also seem unfair and unrealistic to expect inmates to earn enough money during their stay in prison, or immediately after their release into the community, so as to be able to pay the often exorbitant amounts imposed on them. Indeed, it would appear a distinct possibility that an inmate would be tempted to resort to illegitimate means to be able to procure such money during his period of incarceration, or worse, after his release from prison. While the author is by no means advocating a lenient stance by our courts when dealing with convicted criminals it is obvious that imposing excessive fines on persons that do not have a reasonable chance of paying them is counterproductive and only leads to a higher burden on the already stretched resources and budget allocated for the Corradino Correctional Facility. Moreover it is a glaring sign of inefficiency and failure of our justice system that an inmate is released from prison only to be sent back after a few months or even years on charges that had been pending for years. Supervised community work and an opportunity to repay reasonable fines through specialised employment schemes would perhaps produce better results for all parties. The Government would do well to address these anomalies in our legal system when it embarks on the much awaited reform of the justice sector.

References

American Psychiatric Association. (2000). *Diagnostic and statistical manual of mental disorders* (4th ed., text rev.). Washington, DC: Author.

American Psychiatric Association. (2013). *Diagnostic and statistical manual of mental disorders* (5th ed.). Washington, DC: Author.

Bureau of Justice Statistics. (1995*). Drugs and crime facts, 1994: A summary of drug data published in 1994.* Washington, DC: Bureau of Justice Statistics.

Burke, A.C. & Gregoire, T.K. (2007). *Substance abuse treatment outcomes for coerced and noncoerced clients.* Health & Social Work, 32(1), 7-15.

Dangerous Drugs Ordinance. In *Laws of Malta*, 1939. Last revised 2009. Retrieved from http://justiceservices.gov.mt/DownloadDocument.aspx?app=lom&itemid=8641&l=1

Dekel, R., Benbenishty, R. & Amran, Y. (2004). *Therapeutic communities for drug addicts: Prediction of long-term outcomes.* Addictive Behaviours, 29, 1833-1837

De Leon G. (2000) *The therapeutic community: Theory, model and method.* New York: Springer Publishing Company.

Eisenberg, M., & Fabelo, T. (1996). *Evaluation of the Texas correctional substance abuse treatment initiative: The impact of policy research.* Crime & Delinquency, 42(2), 296-308.

European Monitoring Centre for Drugs and Drug Addiction. (2011). *Annual report 2011: the state of the drugs problem in Europe.* Luxembourg: Publications Office of the European Union. Retrieved from http://www.emcdda.europa.eu/attachements.cfm/att_143743_EN_EMCDDA_AR201 1_EN.pdf

European Monitoring Centre for Drugs and Drug Addiction. (2012). *Annual report 2012: the state of the drugs problem in Europe*. Luxembourg: Publications Office of the European Union. Retrieved from http://www.emcdda.europa.eu/attachements.cfm/att_190854_EN_TDAC12001ENC_.pdf

Foundation for Social Welfare Services (2011). *2007-2009 Report*. Santa Venera, Malta: Author. Retrieved from https://secure3.gov.mt/socialpolicy/admin/contentlibrary/Uploads/MediaFile/fsws_operations_report.pdf

Gellel, M., Olivari D'Emanuele, C. & Muscat, R. (2011). *Malta drug situation 2008-2010 national report*. Ministry of Education, Employment and the Family, Valletta. Malta. Retrieved from http://www.doi-archived.gov.mt/EN/press_releases/2011/12/pr2426a.pdf

Gendreau, P., Little, T., & Goggin, C. (1996). *A meta-analysis of the predictors of adult offender recidivism: What works!* Criminology, 34(4), 575–607.

Gossop, M., Trakada, K., Stewart, D. & Witton, J. (2005). *Reductions in criminal convictions after addiction treatment: 5-year follow-up*. Drug and Alcohol Dependence, 79, 295-302.

Griffith, J.D., Hiller, M.L., Knight, K., & Simpson, D.D. (1999). *A cost-effectiveness analysis of in-prison therapeutic community treatment and risk classification*. The Prison Journal, 79(3), 352-368.

Hall, E.A., Prendergast, M.L., Wellisch, J., Patten, M., & Cao, Y. (2004). *Treating drugabusing women prisoners: An outcomes evaluation of the Forever Free Program*. The Prison Journal, 84(1), 81-105.

Hibell, B., Guttormsson, U., Ahlström, S., Balakireva, O., Bjarnason, T., Kokkevi, A., Kraus, L. (2012), *The 2011 ESPAD report. Substance use among students in 36 European countries.* The Swedish Council for Information on Alcohol and Other Drugs, Stockholm, Sweden. Retrieved from http://www.espad.org/Uploads/ESPAD_reports/2011/The_2011_ESPAD_Report_FULL_2012_10_29.pdf

Hiller, M.L., Knight, K., & Simpson, D.D. (1999). *Prison-based substance abuse treatment, residential aftercare and recidivism.* Addiction, 94(6), 833-842.

Horney, J., Osgood, D. W., & Marshall, I. H. (1995). *Criminal careers in the short-term: Intra-individual variability in crime and its relation to local life circumstances.* American Sociological Review, 60, 655–673

Inciardi, J.A. & Martin, S.S. (1993). *Drug abuse treatment in criminal justice settings. Journal of Drug Issues,* 23(1), 1-6.

Inciardi, J.A., Martin, S.S., Butzin, C.A., Hooper, R.M. & Harrison, L.D. (1997). *An effective model of prison-based treatment for drug-involved offenders.* Journal of Drug Issues, 27(2), 261-278.

Inciardi, J.A., Martin, S.S., & Butzin, C.A. (2004). *Five-year outcomes of therapeutic community treatment of drug-involved offenders after release from prison.* Crime & Delinquency, 50(1), 88-107.

Knight, K., Simpson, D.D., & Hiller, M. (1999). *Three-year reincarceration outcomes for in-prison therapeutic community treatment in Texas.* The Prison Journal, 79(3), 337-351.

Landenberger, N.A. & Lipsey, M.W. (2005). *The positive effects of cognitive-behavioral programs for offenders: A meta-analysis of factors associated with effective treatment.* Journal of Experimental Criminology, 1(4), 451-476.

Langan, N.P. & Pelissier, B.M.M. (2001). *The effect of drug treatment on inmate misconduct in federal prisons.* Journal of Offender Rehabilitation, 34(2), 21-30.

MacKenzie, D. L., Browning, K., Skroban, S. S., & Smith, D. A. (1999). *The impact of probation on the criminal activities of offenders.* Journal of Research in Crime and Delinquency, 36(4), 423–453.

Malinowski, A. (2003). *'What works' with substance users in prison?* Journal of Substance Use, 8(4), 223-233.

Malta. Parliament. House of Representatives. (2011). Questions, 11th Legislature, Session 307, (23092).

Martin, S.S., Butzin, C.A., Saum, C.A., & Inciardi, J.A. (1999). *Three-year outcomes of therapeutic community treatment for drug-involved offenders in Delaware: From prison to work release to aftercare.* The Prison Journal, 79(3), 294-320.

McMurran, M. (2007). *What works in substance misuse treatments for offenders?* Criminal Behaviour and Mental Health, 17, 225-233.

Medical and Kindred Professions Ordinance. In *Laws of Malta,* 1901. Last revised 2012. Retrieved from http://justiceservices.gov.mt/DownloadDocument.aspx?app=lom&itemid=8591&l=1

Messina, N., Burdon, W., Hagopian, J.D., & Prendergast, M. (2006). *Predictors of prison-based treatment outcomes: A comparison of men and women participants.* The American Journal of Drug and Alcohol Abuse, 32, 7-28

Mitchell, O., Wilson, D. B., & MacKenzie, D. L. (2007). *Does incarceration-based drug treatment reduce recidivism? A metaanalytic synthesis of the research.* Journal of Experimental Criminology, 3(4), 353-375.

Miller, Patrice M. (2010). *The Impact of Prison-based Substance Abuse Treatment on Rates of Recidivism among Female Offenders.* Ph.D. dissertation, Capella University. Retrieved from ProQuest Dissertations & Theses Database, 3404637

Mosher, C. & Phillips, D. (2006). *The dynamics of prison-based therapeutic community for women offenders.* The Prison Journal, 86(1), 6-31.

National Statistics Office. (2009). Lifestyle Survey 2007. Malta: Author. Retrieved from http://www.nso.gov.mt/statdoc/document_file.aspx?id=2483

Pearson, F.S. & Lipton, D.S. (1999). *A meta-analytic review of the effectiveness of corrections-based treatment for drug abuse.* The Prison Journal, 79(4), 384-410.

Pearson, F.S., Lipton, D.S., Cleland, C.M., & Yee, D.S. (2002). *The effects of behavioral/cognitive-behavioral programs on recisivism.* Crime & Delinquency, 48(3), 476-49

Pelissier, B., Rhodes, W., Saylor, W., Gaes, G., Camp, S.D., Vanyur, S.D. et al. (2001). *Triad drug treatment evaluation project.* Federal Probation, 65(3), 3-7.

Pelissier, B., Motivans, M., & Rounds-Bryant, J.L. (2005). *Substance abuse treatment outcomes: A multi-site study of male and female prison programs.* Journal of Offender Rehabilitation, 41(2), 57-80.

Pollock, J. M. (2004). *Prisons and prison life: Costs and consequences.* Los Angeles: Roxbury.

Prendergast, M., Farabee, D., & Cartier, J. (2001). *The impact of in-prison therapeutic community programs on prison management.* Journal of Offender Rehabilitation, 32(3), 63-78.

Prendergast, M.L., Hall, E.A., & Wexler, H.K. (2003*). Multiple measures of outcome in assessing a prison-based drug treatment program.* Journal of Offender Rehabilitation,

37(3- 4), 65-94.

Prendergast, M.L., Podus, D., Chang, E., & Urada, D. (2002). *The effectiveness of drug abuse treatment: a meta-analysis of comparison group studies*. Drug and Alcohol Dependence, 67(1), 53 - 72.

Prendergast, M.L., Hall, E.A., Wexler, H.K., Melnick, G. & Cao, Y. (2004). *Amity prison-based therapeutic community: 5-year outcomes*. The Prison Journal, 84(1), 36-60.

Quinones, M.A.; Doyle, K.M.; Sheffet, A.; and Louria, D.B. (1979*) Evaluation of drug abuse rehabilitation efforts: A review*. Am J Pub Health, 69(11): 1164-1169

Substance Abuse and Mental Health Services Administration (2005). *Substance abuse treatment for adults in the criminal justice system. Treatment Improvement Protocol (TIP)* Series 44. DHHS Publication No. (SMA) 05-4056. Rockville, MD.

Taxman, F.S. & Bouffard, J.A. (2002). *Assessing therapeutic integrity in modified therapeutic communities for drug-involved offenders*. The Prison Journal, 82(2), 189-212.

Welsh, W, N., (2009). *A Multi-Site Evaluation of Prison-Based Drug Treatment: A Research Partnership Between The Pennsylvania Department of Corrections and Temple University - Final Report to the Pennsylvania Commission on Crime and Delinquency.* Temple University. Philadelphia. Retrieved from http://www.portal.state.pa.us/portal/server.pt/document/882761/multi-site_evaluation_of_prison-based_drug_treatment_final_report_pdf+&cd=1&hl=en&ct=clnk&gl=mt

Wexler, H.K., DeLeon, G., Thomas, G., Kressel, D. & Peters, J. (1999). *The Amity prison TC evaluation: Reincarceration Outcomes.* Criminal Justice and Behavior,

26(2), 147-167.

World Health Organization. (2008). *ICD-10: International statistical classification of diseases and related health problems* (10th Rev. ed.). New York, NY: Author.

Ziegler, R., Kohutek, K., & Owen, P. (1978). *A multimodal treatment approach for incarcerated alcoholics.* Journal of Clinical Psychology, 34(4), 1005-1009.

Appendix A: Statistical tables used in Research Question Number One

Table A1

Cross tabulation of study participants by sex

			GROUP			
			1	2	3	Total
SEX[a]	1	Count	27	213	98	338
		% within SEX	8.0%	63.0%	29.0%	100.0%
		% within GROUP	100.0%	93.0%	93.3%	93.6%
		% of Total	7.5%	59.0%	27.1%	93.6%
	2	Count	0	16	7	23
		% within SEX	.0%	69.6%	30.4%	100.0%
		% within GROUP	.0%	7.0%	6.7%	6.4%
		% of Total	.0%	4.4%	1.9%	6.4%
Total		Count	27	229	105	361
		% within SEX	7.5%	63.4%	29.1%	100.0%
		% within GROUP	100.0%	100.0%	100.0%	100.0%
		% of Total	7.5%	63.4%	29.1%	100.0%

a. 1 = males, 2 = females

Table A2

Descriptive statistics of study participants by age on admission

					95% Confidence Interval for Mean			
GRP	N	Mean	Std. Deviation	Std. Error	Lower Bound	Upper Bound	Minimum	Maximum
1	27	29.85	5.875	1.131	27.53	32.18	19	42
2	229	29.50	9.150	.605	28.31	30.69	14	59
3	105	28.21	7.396	.722	26.78	29.64	16	50
Total	361	29.15	8.467	.446	28.28	30.03	14	59

Table A3
Descriptive statistics of study participants by age at first conviction

GRP	N	Mean	Std. Deviation	Std. Error	95% Confidence Interval for Mean		Minimum	Maximum
					Lower Bound	Upper Bound		
1	27	25.11	5.147	.990	23.08	27.15	17	34
2	229	27.31	7.963	.526	26.27	28.34	14	59
3	105	24.46	5.852	.571	23.32	25.59	15	41
Total	361	26.31	7.329	.386	25.55	27.07	14	59

Table A4
Cross tabulation of study participants by occupation

			GROUP			
			1	2	3	Total
OCC[a]	0	Count	26	177	82	285
		% within GRP	96.3%	77.3%	78.1%	78.9%
		% of Total	7.2%	49.0%	22.7%	78.9%
	1	Count	1	52	23	76
		% within GRP	3.7%	22.7%	21.9%	21.1%
		% of Total	.3%	14.4%	6.4%	21.1%
Total		Count	27	229	105	361
		% within GRP	100.0%	100.0%	100.0%	100.0%
		% of Total	7.5%	63.4%	29.1%	100.0%

a.0 = unemployed, 1 = employed

Table A5

Cross tabulation of study participants by recidivism

			GRP			
			1	2	3	Total
REOFF[a]	0	Count	8	132	47	187
		% within GRP	29.6%	57.6%	44.8%	51.8%
		% of Total	2.2%	36.6%	13.0%	51.8%
	1	Count	19	97	58	174
		% within GRP	70.4%	42.4%	55.2%	48.2%
		% of Total	5.3%	26.9%	16.1%	48.2%
Total		Count	27	229	105	361
		% within GRP	100.0%	100.0%	100.0%	100.0%
		% of Total	7.5%	63.4%	29.1%	100.0%

a.0 = Did not reoffend, 1 = Reoffended

Table A6

Cross tabulation of study participants by profile of offence on admission

| | | | GROUP | | | |
			1	2	3	Total
Offence on Admission	Property	Count	13	75	62	150
		% within GROUP	48.1%	32.8%	59.0%	41.6%
		% of Total	3.6%	20.8%	17.2%	41.6%
	Person	Count	3	21	9	33
		% within GROUP	11.1%	9.2%	8.6%	9.1%
		% of Total	.8%	5.8%	2.5%	9.1%
	ConvAdmn[a]	Count	2	27	3	32
		% within GROUP	7.4%	11.8%	2.9%	8.9%
		% of Total	.6%	7.5%	.8%	8.9%
	BreachCourt[b]	Count	2	20	2	24
		% within GROUP	7.4%	8.7%	1.9%	6.6%
		% of Total	.6%	5.5%	.6%	6.6%
	Others	Count	1	4	1	6
		% within GROUP	3.7%	1.7%	1.0%	1.7%
		% of Total	.3%	1.1%	.3%	1.7%
	Drugs	Count	6	82	28	116
		% within GROUP	22.2%	35.8%	26.7%	32.1%
		% of Total	1.7%	22.7%	7.8%	32.1%
Total		Count	27	229	105	361
		% within GROUP	100.0%	100.0%	100.0%	100.0%
		% of Total	7.5%	63.4%	29.1%	100.0%

a. conversion of administrative fines into custodial sentences
b. breach of court-imposed conditions

71

Table A7

Cross tabulation of study participants by profile of re-offences

			GROUP			
			1	2	3	Total
Re-offences	Property	Count	10	37	37	84
		% within GRP	52.6%	38.1%	63.8%	48.3%
	Person	Count	2	7	3	12
		% within GRP	10.5%	7.2%	5.2%	6.9%
	ConvAdmn[a]	Count	2	29	10	41
		% within GRP	10.5%	29.9%	17.2%	23.6%
	BreachCourt[b]	Count	2	6	2	10
		% within GRP	10.5%	6.2%	3.4%	5.7%
	Others	Count	1	3	1	5
		% within GRP	5.3%	3.1%	1.7%	2.9%
	Drugs	Count	2	15	5	22
		% within GRP	10.5%	15.5%	8.6%	12.6%
Total		Count	19	97	58	174
		% within GRP	100.0%	100.0%	100.0%	100.0%

a. conversion of administrative fines into custodial sentences

b. breach of court-imposed conditions

Table A8

Cross tabulation of study participants by number of previous convictions

			GROUP			
			1	2	3	Total
PREV[a]	0	Count	12	171	54	237
		% within PREV	5.1%	72.2%	22.8%	100.0%
	1	Count	3	18	22	43
		% within PREV	7.0%	41.9%	51.2%	100.0%
	2	Count	7	16	9	32
		% within PREV	21.9%	50.0%	28.1%	100.0%
	3	Count	5	24	20	49
		% within PREV	10.2%	49.0%	40.8%	100.0%
Total		Count	27	229	105	361
		% within PREV	7.5%	63.4%	29.1%	100.0%

a.Number of previous convictions: : 0 = no previous convictions, 1 = one
previous conviction, 2 = two previous convictions and 3+ = three or more
previous convictions

Table A9

Cross tabulation of study participants by in-prison replacement treatment

			GROUP			
			1	2	3	Total
REPL[a]	0	Count	5	84	17	106
		% within REPL	4.7%	79.2%	16.0%	100.0%
	1	Count	2	25	10	37
		% within REPL	5.4%	67.6%	27.0%	100.0%
	2	Count	20	120	78	218
		% within REPL	9.2%	55.0%	35.8%	100.0%
Total		Count	27	229	105	361
		% within REPL	7.5%	63.4%	29.1%	100.0%

a.In-prison replacement treatment: 0=no replacement treatment, 1=on tramadol
only, 2=on methadone treatment with or without tramadol

Table A10

Cross tabulation of study participants by in-prison psychiatric treatment

			GROUP 1	2	3	Total
PSY[a]	0	Count	3	70	11	84
		% within PSY	3.6%	83.3%	13.1%	100.0%
	1	Count	24	159	94	277
		% within PSY	8.7%	57.4%	33.9%	100.0%
Total		Count	27	229	105	361
		% within PSY	7.5%	63.4%	29.1%	100.0%

a.In-Prison Psychiatric Treatment: 0=no psychiatric treatment, 1=on psychiatric treatment

Table A11

Fisher's Exact Test - Difference between groups with regard to sex

	Value	df	Asymp. Sig. (2-sided)	Exact Sig. (2-sided)	Exact Sig. (1-sided)	Point Probability
Likelihood Ratio	3.711	2	.156	.264		
Fisher's Exact Test	1.552			.537		
Linear-by-Linear Association		1	.439	.452	.279	.113
N of Valid Cases	361					

Table A12

ANOVA - Difference between groups with regard to age on admission

	Sum of Squares	df	Mean Square	F	Sig.
Between Groups	134.574	2	67.287	.938	.392
Within Groups	25676.047	358	71.721		
Total	25810.620	360			

Table A13

Chi-Square Tests - Difference between groups with regard to occupation

	Value	df	Asymp. Sig. (2-sided)
Pearson Chi-Square	5.313	2	.070
Likelihood Ratio	7.270	2	.026
Linear-by-Linear Association	1.622	1	.203
N of Valid Cases	361		

Table A14

Chi-Square Tests - Difference between groups with regard to the number of previous convictions

	Value	df	Asymp. Sig. (2-sided)
Pearson Chi-Square	32.505[a]	6	.000
Likelihood Ratio	28.823	6	.000
Linear-by-Linear Association	1.242	1	.265
N of Valid Cases	361		

a. 3 cells (25.0%) have expected count less than 5. The minimum expected count is 2.39.

Table A15

Chi-Square Tests - Difference between groups with regard to in-prison replacement treatment

	Value	df	Asymp. Sig. (2-sided)
Pearson Chi-Square	18.444[a]	4	.001
Likelihood Ratio	19.364	4	.001
Linear-by-Linear Association	5.137	1	.023
N of Valid Cases	361		

a. 1 cells (11.1%) have expected count less than 5. The minimum expected count is 2.77.

Table A16

Chi-Square Tests - Difference between groups with regard to in-prison psychiatric treatment

	Value	df	Asymp. Sig. (2-sided)
Pearson Chi-Square	18.692[a]	2	.000
Likelihood Ratio	20.468	2	.000
Linear-by-Linear Association	4.997	1	.025
N of Valid Cases	361		

a. 0 cells (.0%) have expected count less than 5. The minimum expected count is 6.28.

Table A17

Chi-Square Tests - Difference between groups with regard to recidivism rates

	Value	df	Asymp. Sig. (2-sided)
Pearson Chi-Square	10.529[a]	2	.005
Likelihood Ratio	10.671	2	.005
Linear-by-Linear Association	.068	1	.794
N of Valid Cases	361		

a. 0 cells (.0%) have expected count less than 5. The minimum expected count is 13.01.

Appendix B: Statistical tables used in Research Question Number Two

Table B1
Cross tabulation of study participants by sex

			GROUP		
			1	2	Total
SEX[a]	1	Count	48	50	98
		% within GROUP	100.0%	87.7%	93.3%
	2	Count	0	7	7
		% within GROUP	.0%	12.3%	6.7%
Total		Count	48	57	105
		% within GROUP	100.0%	100.0%	100.0%

a. 1 = males, 2 = females

Table B2
Descriptive statistics of study participants by age on admission

	GRP	N	Mean	Std. Deviation	Std. Error Mean
AGE	1	48	28.92	7.040	1.016
	2	57	27.61	7.695	1.019

Table B3
Descriptive statistics of study participants by age at first conviction

	GRP	N	Mean	Std. Deviation	Std. Error Mean
AGE1st	1	48	25.23	5.688	.821
	2	57	23.81	5.960	.789

Table B4

Crosstabulation of study participants by occupation

			GROUP		
			1	2	Total
OCC[a]	0	Count	32	50	82
		% within GRP	66.7%	87.7%	78.1%
	1	Count	16	7	23
		% within GRP	33.3%	12.3%	21.9%
Total		Count	48	57	105
		% within GRP	100.0%	100.0%	100.0%

a.0 = unemployed, 1 = employed

Table B5

Cross tabulation of study participants by recidivism

			GROUP		
			1	2	Total
REOFF[a]	0	Count	26	21	47
		% within GROUP	54.2%	36.8%	44.8%
	1	Count	22	36	58
		% within GROUP	45.8%	63.2%	55.2%
Total		Count	48	57	105
		% within GROUP	100.0%	100.0%	100.0%

a.0 = Did not reoffend, 1 = Reoffended

Table B6

Cross tabulation of study participants by profile of offence on admission

			GROUP		Total
			1	2	
Offence on Admission	Property	Count	27	35	62
		% within GROUP	56.3%	61.4%	59.0%
	Person	Count	2	7	9
		% within GROUP	4.2%	12.3%	8.6%
	ConvAdmn[a]	Count	2	1	3
		% within GROUP	4.2%	1.8%	2.9%
	BreachCourt[b]	Count	0	2	2
		% within GROUP	.0%	3.5%	1.9%
	Others	Count	0	1	1
		% within GROUP	.0%	1.8%	1.0%
	Drugs	Count	17	11	28
		% within GROUP	35.4%	19.3%	26.7%
Total		Count	48	57	105
		% within GROUP	100.0%	100.0%	100.0%

a. conversion of administrative fines into custodial sentences

b. breach of court-imposed conditions

Table B7

Cross tabulation of study participants by profile of re-offences

			GROUP		Total
			1	2	
Re-offences	Property	Count	16	21	37
		% within GROUP	72.7%	58.3%	63.8%
	Person	Count	0	3	3
		% within GROUP	.0%	8.3%	5.2%
	ConvAdmn[a]	Count	6	4	10
		% within GROUP	27.3%	11.1%	17.2%
	BreachCourt[b]	Count	0	2	2
		% within GROUP	.0%	5.6%	3.4%
	Others	Count	0	1	1
		% within GROUP	.0%	2.8%	1.7%
	Drugs	Count	0	5	5
		% within GROUP	.0%	13.9%	8.6%
Total		Count	22	36	58
		% within GROUP	100.0%	100.0%	100.0%

a. conversion of administrative fines into custodial sentences

b. breach of court-imposed conditions

Table B8

Cross tabulation of study participants (sorted by prison inmate program) by recidivism

			Prison Inmate Program (PiP)			Total
			1[b]	2[c]	3[d]	
REOFF[a]	0	Count	13	18	16	47
		% within PiP	40.6%	51.4%	42.1%	44.8%
	1	Count	19	17	22	58
		% within PiP	59.4%	48.6%	57.9%	55.2%
Total		Count	32	35	38	105
		% within PiP	100.0%	100.0%	100.0%	100.0%

a.0 = Did not reoffend, 1 = Reoffended

b. SATU

c. SEDQA

d. CARITAS

Table B9

Cross tabulation of study participants by number of previous convictions

			GROUP		
			1	2	Total
PREV[a]	0	Count	29	25	54
		% within GROUP	60.4%	43.9%	51.4%
	1	Count	7	15	22
		% within GROUP	14.6%	26.3%	21.0%
	2	Count	3	6	9
		% within GROUP	6.3%	10.5%	8.6%
	3	Count	9	11	20
		% within GROUP	18.8%	19.3%	19.0%
Total		Count	48	57	105
		% within GROUP	100.0%	100.0%	100.0%

a.Number of previous convictions: : 0 = no previous convictions, 1 = one previous conviction, 2 = two previous convictions and 3+ = three or more previous convictions

Table B10

Cross tabulation of study participants by in-prison replacement treatment

			GRP		Total
			1	2	
REPL[a]	0	Count	4	5	9
		% within GROUP	8.3%	8.8%	8.6%
	1	Count	2	1	3
		% within GROUP	4.2%	1.8%	2.9%
	2	Count	42	51	93
		% within G GROUP	87.5%	89.5%	88.6%
Total		Count	48	57	105
		% within GROUP	100.0%	100.0%	100.0%

a.In-prison replacement treatment: 0=no replacement treatment, 1=on tramadol only, 2=on methadone treatment with or without tramadol

Table B11

Cross tabulation of study participants by in-prison psychiatric treatment

			GRP		Total
			1	2	
PSY[a]	0	Count	10	1	11
		% within GRP	20.8%	1.8%	10.5%
	1	Count	38	56	94
		% within GRP	79.2%	98.2%	89.5%
Total		Count	48	57	105
		% within GRP	100.0%	100.0%	100.0%

a.In-Prison Psychiatric Treatment: 0=no psychiatric treatment, 1=on psychiatric treatment

Table B12
Fisher's Exact Test - Difference between groups with regard to sex

	Value	df	Asymp. Sig. (2-sided)	Exact Sig. (2-sided)	Exact Sig. (1-sided)
Pearson Chi-Square	6.316[a]	1	.012		
Continuity Correction[b]	4.496	1	.034		
Likelihood Ratio	8.973	1	.003		
Fisher's Exact Test				.015	.012
Linear-by-Linear Association	6.256	1	.012		
N of Valid Cases	105				

a. 2 cells (50.0%) have expected count less than 5. The minimum expected count is 3.20.
b. Computed only for a 2x2 table

Table B13
Chi-Square Tests - Difference between groups with regard to occupation

	Value	df	Asymp. Sig. (2-sided)	Exact Sig. (2-sided)	Exact Sig. (1-sided)
Pearson Chi-Square	6.751[a]	1	.009		
Continuity Correction[b]	5.577	1	.018		
Likelihood Ratio	6.829	1	.009		
Fisher's Exact Test				.017	.009
Linear-by-Linear Association	6.687	1	.010		
N of Valid Cases	105				

a. 0 cells (.0%) have expected count less than 5. The minimum expected count is 10.51.
b. Computed only for a 2x2 table

Table B14

Independent Samples Test - Difference between groups with regard to age on admission

		Levene's Test for Equality of Variances		t-test for Equality of Means				
		F	Sig.	t	df	Sig. (2-tailed)	Mean Difference	Std. Error Difference
AGE	Equal variances assumed	.055	.814	.898	103	.371	1.303	1.450
	Equal variances not assumed			.905	102.27	.368	1.303	1.439

Table B15

Independent Samples Test - Difference between groups with regard to age at first conviction

		Levene's Test for Equality of Variances		t-test for Equality of Means				
		F	Sig.	t	df	Sig. (2-tailed)	Mean Difference	Std. Error Difference
AGE 1st	Equal variances assumed	.144	.705	1.244	103	.216	1.422	1.143
	Equal variances not assumed			1.249	101.36	.215	1.422	1.139

Table B16

Chi-Square Tests - Difference between groups with regard to the number of previous convictions

	Value	df	Asymp. Sig. (2-sided)
Pearson Chi-Square	3.661[a]	3	.300
Likelihood Ratio	3.721	3	.293
Linear-by-Linear Association	.913	1	.339
N of Valid Cases	105		

a. 2 cells (25.0%) have expected count less than 5. The minimum expected count is 4.11.

Table B17

Chi-Square Tests - Difference between groups with regard to in-prison replacement treatment

	Value	df	Asymp. Sig. (2-sided)
Pearson Chi-Square	.548[a]	2	.760
Likelihood Ratio	.551	2	.759
Linear-by-Linear Association	.018	1	.892
N of Valid Cases	105		

a. 4 cells (66.7%) have expected count less than 5. The minimum expected count is 1.37.

Table B18
Chi-Square Tests - Difference between groups with regard to in-prison psychiatric treatment

	Value	df	Asymp. Sig. (2-sided)	Exact Sig. (2-sided)	Exact Sig. (1-sided)
Pearson Chi-Square	10.113[a]	1	.001		
Continuity Correction[b]	8.181	1	.004		
Likelihood Ratio	11.243	1	.001		
Fisher's Exact Test				.002	.002
Linear-by-Linear Association	10.017	1	.002		
N of Valid Cases	105				

a. 0 cells (.0%) have expected count less than 5. The minimum expected count is 5.03.
b. Computed only for a 2x2 table

Table B19
Chi-Square Tests - Difference between programs with regard to recidivism rates

	Value	df	Asymp. Sig. (2-sided)
Pearson Chi-Square	.959[a]	2	.619
Likelihood Ratio	.957	2	.620
Linear-by-Linear Association	.006	1	.940
N of Valid Cases	105		

a. 0 cells (.0%) have expected count less than 5. The minimum expected count is 14.32.

Table B20

Chi-Square Tests- Difference between groups with regard to recidivism rates

	Value	df	Asymp. Sig. (2-sided)	Exact Sig. (2-sided)	Exact Sig. (1-sided)
Pearson Chi-Square	3.163[a]	1	.075		
Continuity Correction[b]	2.501	1	.114		
Likelihood Ratio	3.173	1	.075		
Fisher's Exact Test				.081	.057
Linear-by-Linear Association	3.133	1	.077		
N of Valid Cases	105				

a. 0 cells (.0%) have expected count less than 5. The minimum expected count is 21.49.

b. Computed only for a 2x2 table